The Analyst and the Adolescent at Work

The Analyst and the Adolescent at Work

Marjorie Harley   Editor

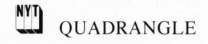 QUADRANGLE

The New York Times Book Co.

Library of Congress Catalog Card Number: 72-91379
International Standard Book Number: 0-8129-0324-2

Contents

Preface

The idea for this book was conceived by Elisabeth Geleerd. Prompted by her desire to provide a lifelike portrayal of the technique of child analysis—one which would convey the child's phase-specific modes of communication and the interplay between child and analyst—Dr. Geleerd conceived and edited *The Child Analyst at Work*. (New York: International Universities Press, 1966). Then she turned her energies toward designing a companion book, which would convey, also through firsthand clinical accounts, both the generic and distinctive features of the analysis of adolescents. But barely had she embarked on this project when death intervened.

At the request of her friends and colleagues, I undertook to carry out Dr. Geleerd's plans for this book. Our wish to complete the task she had set for herself had a twofold source: we wished the finished book to represent a tribute to Elisabeth Geleerd and we believed in the intrinsic value of such a book for those engaged in the analysis of adolescents and in related fields of work.

Dr. Geleerd had discussed with me—albeit in rough and rapid outline—her hope to produce a book of this nature and had mentioned that she would not insist (as she had when preparing her first book) on the inclusion of so many detailed descriptions of individual analytic sessions. It was my impression that she was keenly aware of the many issues pertaining to the analysis of adolescents and thus wished to allow room for discussion of any such issues as the authors might want to consider. I believed, therefore, that I was acting in accord with Dr. Geleerd's intent when I offered this leeway to the contributors. In other respects, I could know only that I was carrying out Dr. Geleerd's purpose in the most general way: that is, to demonstrate to the reader, through the medium of a variety of clinical papers, that the method of classical psychoanalysis might be successfully applied in the treatment of adolescents and to illustrate some of the ways in which this method might be implemented.

If this book succeeds in these two aims, the credit is Elisabeth Geleerd's. But responsibility for any and all flaws in selection, arrangement, and editing is mine alone.

Introduction

Marjorie Harley   *Baltimore*

This book is concerned with the psychoanalytic treatment of adolescents. Each contributor was asked to write a clinical paper which would discuss the course and vicissitudes of an individual analysis or which would scrutinize a particular clinical problem illustrated by a given analysis.

As I read these papers, I found that they reflected a wide range of focal interests and varying degrees and kinds of psychopathology. From this angle, it seemed that each paper would have to be taken separately and there would be little that would lend itself to a unified whole. But when I looked at things from a different perspective and asked myself what the purpose of this book was in the first place, I concluded that this diversity might prove more of an asset than a liability.

It is a matter of common knowledge that analysts are of more than one mind in respect to the suitability of the psychoanalytic method for the treatment of adolescents. Some consider few if any adolescent patients analyzable without recourse to all manner of parameters or modifications of technique which are incompatible with the analytic method itself. Others restrict their criteria for analyzability to those adolescents with "classical neuroses" rooted in and centered around oedipal conflicts. Finally, there are those analysts who believe that the analytic treatment method is applicable to a somewhat wider spectrum of pathological formations in adolescents. It is evident that by and large the papers in this book reflect this last viewpoint.

A number of factors doubtless contribute to the disparity of opinion regarding the analyzability of adolescents. Although I cannot here enumerate all of these, foremost among them are the oft-repeated descriptions of the turbulence wrought by the special nature of the developmental processes of this period: the impact of the increased force of the drives with the concomitant ego-id imbalances and the enhanced proclivity for acting out; the partial structural dissolutions and consequent structural fluidity; the marked threat of regressive pulls; the withdrawal of cathexis from the infantile love objects; the intensification of narcissism; and the not infrequent lowered level of self-esteem which lessens the capacity for realistic self-appraisal. These are but some of the well known aspects of adolescence and few if any analysts would question their validity. When viewed collectively, however, they would seem to underscore unavoidable and well-nigh insurmountable obstacles to the unfolding of an ongoing analytic process and a workable transference.

But although in one sense justifiable, such global statements about adolescence present us with a composite picture which may tend to obscure individual differences and to promote a kind of stereotyped version of what an adolescent is. No doubt there are some adolescents who come close to approximating this composite picture. Yet in our work with individual adolescents rarely do we find all these obstacles operating simultaneously and in equal measure within a single patient. For example, developmental lags as well as the dynamic interplay between regressive and progressive forces may yield an assortment of structural imbalances and counter-balances which vary from individual to individual. Or, in accordance with the character of his defensive system—its strength, rigidity or friability—the adolescent may appear to function relatively smoothly, he may be inhibited and withdrawn, or he may engage in acting out of greater or less severity.

Furthermore, these sometimes rather sweeping generalizations about adolescents do not always take into account the differences between the sub-phases of adolescence:[1] that is, the phase-specific developmental tasks and phase-specific conflicts of the pre-adolescent are not the same as those of the early adolescent; and both the pre-adolescent and the early adolescent are characterized by features in many respects different from those which distinguish later adolescence. There are in fact as many individual variations among the adolescents who enter our consulting rooms as there are among those child and adult patients whom we encounter. This assertion is not intended to negate the validity and value of the aforementioned conceptualizations of adolescent development. It is merely meant to suggest that from the clinical vantage, although these conceptualizations contribute enormously to our assessment and understanding of all adolescents, we should not apply them in a way such as to lose sight of fundamental individual differences. It was this matter of individual variations which led me to conclude that the diversification afforded by the papers in this book might be advantageous.

These papers touch upon many areas of interest, each of which could provide sufficient subject matter for further study and scrutiny. I shall remark on only a few of those points which to my mind are either implicit or explicit in most if not all of the individual contributions.

To begin with, there is the question of the extent to which a workable transference may develop in adolescence and the degree to which this may be utilized for the analytic work. Opposing views have been expressed by a number of analysts in respect to the role of transference in the analysis of adolescents. It is especially in the case of the younger adolescent that many believe the prevalent concern with daily activities revolving around peer life and the concomitant need to detach oneself from the infantile love objects, prevent the development of transference, or dilute it, or impede its accessibility to interpretation.

It is therefore significant to note how frequently a workable transference manifested itself in the analyses described in this book and how more than one author demonstrated through the actual clinical material the formation of a transference neurosis.

Although the majority of contributors appear to have accepted the role of transference in the analyses of adolescents as a matter of course, Carl Adatto notes that he has often encountered a marked decrease in the potential for analyzing the transference of adolescent patients, particularly after a period of intensive and fruitful analytic work has taken place. He goes on to say, however, that these observations may be peculiar to the kinds of adolescents who have come his way and that they may be representative of "the exception rather than the rule."

I believe we must repeatedly remind ourselves that even within the span of a lifetime, any single analyst can have attained only relatively few first-hand experiences and the part played by transference in the analyses of adolescents is undeniably still an unsettled but crucial issue.[2] It will probably remain so until we have pooled observations from many more cases and further refined our techniques to the point where we may more accurately assess whether the absence or presence of a workable transference, and the extent to which it may develop, are traceable to the distinctive adolescent configurations of each case or to the degree of our ability to perceive various transference manifestations and to deal with them.

Several authors draw our attention to the importance of physio-biological factors in adolescence. Marjorie Sprince emphasizes the universal impact of the physiological changes of puberty and adolescence. Jules Glenn's paper, which centers around the role of masturbation in adolescence, addresses itself specifically to these physio-biological factors and discusses the "actual neurosis" in the light of the "physiological concomitants of sexual excitement." Both Elizabeth Daunton and Marie McCann demonstrate how the physiological changes of puberty favored the analyses of their patients' bisexual conflicts: in the first instance, by bringing the patient's castration material into foreground; in the second, by lessening the prepubertal bisexual confusions and augmenting the patient's desire to accept her own sexual identity.[3] I may well risk stating a truism when I say that the analysis of adolescents illumi-nates with special clarity the essential connections between physio-biological and psychological processes.

One can scarcely mention the analysis of adolescents without commenting on the matter of *adaptations* of technique which are to be sharply differentiated from *parameters* or *modifications* of technique. These adaptations are designed to implement the psychoanalytic method while adhering to the clinical concepts and principles on which this method is based. On the other hand, parameters are incompatible with the psychoanalytic method and, subject to their nature and degree, may contaminate the transfer-ence, and obstruct or even disrupt the analytic process.

Those adaptations of technique which are devised for the analysis of adolescents are governed by a sensitivity to the patient's phase-specific as well as genetically determined areas of ego vulnerabilities and structural conflicts, and by a continuing alertness to the qualitative and quantitative factors in his ego-id balances at any given moment. Technical adaptations demand sufficient flexibility to allow for optimal means of communication from the vantage of both mode and content. They arise from the analyst's understanding of adolescent development as well as of the ways in which the patient's earlier developmental successes or failures—progressions or arrests—may be affecting his manner of coping with his current developmental tasks or may have con-tributed to primary ego deficits. Any such existing ego deficits may be exacerbated but are not ultimately explainable by the adolescent developmental processes and conflicts.

I would tentatively suggest that the differing views of the analyzability of adolescents and their capacity for transference developments may be resolved, at least partially, through further study of an experimentation with a variety of such technical adaptations that adhere to the psychoanalytic method. In this respect, Calvin Settlage's paper is a case in point.

Settlage directs our attention to the fact that the premises for our technical adaptations reside in psychoanalytic ego psychology and he presents us with conceptualizations of the principles underlying a number of techniques which he has designed for the purpose of defense analysis and which involve an awareness of the adolescent's frequent and well-founded need for some defensive reinforcement.[4] With scientific cautiousness, he emphasizes that these techniques should be applied selectively and that they are not applicable to all adolescents, thereby also reminding us that we should always be guided by the needs of a particular adolescent and that we should constantly bear in mind the differences between adolescents.

At this juncture it may be pertinent to remark on the use of parameters (as opposed to technical adaptations) which three of the authors resorted to in the analyses of their patients.

In line with Kurt Eissler's (1953) observations, Marjorie Sprince stresses that the necessity for the introduction of parameters is a "pointer" to the severity of the patient's psychopathology. She further indicates how she introduced a parameter with her patient only after all manner of interpretations had failed and after she had concluded that it was unavoidable because of the special character of the patient's ego deficits.

Moses Laufer chose his patient, also one whose psychopathology was of a severe order, to illustrate his thesis that the analyst may need to adopt a parameter when a seriously disturbed adolescent threatens to endanger his own life or otherwise engage in actions which may harm himself. He describes in dynamic terms why he injected a *temporary* parameter into the treatment of a suicidal girl by setting a limit to her acting out of a central masturbation conflict. This manoeuver enabled the patient to bring the conflict into the analysis. But Laufer goes on to underscore that, with the exception of this single parameter, he believes that a "classical" technique was not only desirable but essential to the attainment of structural changes in his patient.

Finally, Carl Adatto, during one phase of his patient's analysis, injected a parameter because of the boy's epilepsy and other extenuating circumstances.

When contemplating the introduction of such modifications of technique, it is important to ask oneself whether a particular parameter is indeed necessary, whether it will facilitate the analysis and be accessible to later interpretation, or whether it may impede the analytic process and even disrupt the analytic treatment. I think few if any analysts would dispute the fact that not all parameters are later analyzable and that when a patient's psychopathology is so severe as to demand repeated parameters, he is plainly unanalyzable—at least at that time. If parameters are frequently introduced, or if even a single parameter, in one or another way of an extreme nature, is utilized, we can no longer appropriately refer to our method of treatment as psychoanalysis.

Sprince, Laufer and Adatto have clearly implied their agreement on this point and have made explicit their view that they regard parameters as the exception rather than the rule in the analysis of adolescents. In addition, Adatto states that rather than compromise his patient's opportunity for further analysis in later adolescence by deviating from analytic technique, he chose a course which resulted in premature termination. In this context, I am reminded again of Kurt Eissler's (1958) caution against employing psychotherapeutic measures with an adolescent for whom psychoanalysis is the treatment of choice. As Eissler puts it, these measures may lead to an alleviation of the adolescent's discomfort, which, in turn, may prevent him from seeking psychoanalysis at a later time. In such instances, then, he may settle for a less than optimal adaptation when he reaches adulthood.

One of the major tasks which confronts psychoanalysts today is that of applying the analytic method to patients—children, adolescents, adults—whose psychopathology encompasses developmental deviations arising from the first years of life, which have resulted in varying degrees of faulty structural development.

In the past we were accustomed to make a simple dichotomy

between the basically intact ego of the ''good neurotic'' and the basically defective ego of the psychotic or pre-psychotic. Our deeper and subtler understanding of the intricacies and complexities inherent in ego psychology, however, has directed our attention increasingly to a broad spectrum of underlying ego deficits which are not secondary to neurotic conflicts but which predate these.

Moreover, we cannot usually regard this or that ego arrest or deviation in isolation since it interacts with and influences other developmental lines. Nor can we divorce such early developmental deviations from later structural conflicts to whose texture and patterning they contribute. These deviations may range from mild to extremely severe and may manifest a greater or less potential for reversibility.

I am not here suggesting that all psychopathological formations determined by early deviational development are amenable to psychoanalytic treatment. But I am in agreement with those who believe that we should extend our criteria for analyzability to patients whose disturbances are not limited to the classical psychoneuroses. I would further underscore that an essential accompaniment to this extension is the continuing delineation of psychoanalysis as a treatment method lest the demarcation line between it and other forms of psychotherapy be blurred. Furthermore, this delineation must be governed by a steadfast fidelity to the analytic method.

In relation to the foregoing, it is significant that many of the papers in this book not only point to the importance of preoedipal determinants of psychopathology but a number of them also make explicit references to primary structural impairment.

Marjorie Sprince speaks of the early and deep ego damage which underlay the regressive features of her patient and she points to the frequent possibility of reversibility, or at least modification, of such early ego damage.

In Elizabeth Daunton's patient, it is not difficult to detect how the twin relationship eventuated in an incompleted separation-individuation phase and in a persistance of primitive identification mechanisms which led to disturbances of body image and an intensification of the bisexual problem.

The two episodes of severe ego regression that Selma Kramer describes in her patient could scarcely have occurred had his ego been that of a "good neurotic." And Paulina Kernberg refers to her patient's fusion of self and object representations and the role of this fusion in her suicidal fantasies.

Calvin Settlage alludes to the integration into our analytic work of the accelerating accumulations of data on early development when he remarks on his reconstruction of the factors in his patient's failure to attain an adequate resolution of the separation-individuation phase. This kind of integration was already forecast by Hartmann (1951) who subscribed to ". . . the essential importance of keeping psychoanalytic technique flexible, especially when we are trying to establish what technique may gain from additional scientific insights . . ." (p. 144).

Elisabeth Geleerd had a keen interest in early development and in ways and means of utilizing newly gained knowledge of developmental processes for our clinical work. I am sure she would concur with Selma Kramer's expressed hope ". . . that the variety of adolescent analyses described in this book may enable us to reconsider [the pessimism in respect to the criteria for analyzability of adolescents] and encourage us to analyze some adolescents who do not fit within the category of the 'normal neurotic,' and whose parents may not impress us most favorably." (This volume, p.190.)

This book has been a long time in the making and I regret that some of the contributors in particular have had to suffer as a consequence. In large measure this delay was unavoidable. Before her death, Elisabeth Geleerd had received only two papers. Many of the contributors I subsequently invited to participate in this undertaking; and there were the inevitable delays, requests for rewriting, and so on. In the light of both the steady influx of knowledge obtained from developmental research and our continuing clinical experience, we frequently find ourselves shifting our angle of vision and sharpening our perspectives with the passage of time. For these reasons, if for no others, I am sure the delay has been frustrating to some of the authors. Doubtless the degree of my regret in respect to each contributor is commensurate with the length of delay which he or she has had to endure.

NOTES

[1]Peter Blos (1962) has discussed these sub-phases in detail.

[2]It is relevant that Elisabeth Geleerd (1967) made a similar comment in respect to child analysis when she stated that: "The whole problem of transference still needs a great deal of reflection, discussion, and clarification among child analysts." (p. 7).

[3]cf. Harley (1961, 1971).

[4]It is interesting to note that Selma Kramer independently employed one of the technical expediencies on which Settlage elaborates: that of facilitating the "distancing" of her patient's ego from threatening material which he had been warding off.

Bibliography

Blos, Peter (1962). *On Adolescence*. New York, International Universities Press.

Eissler, Kurt R. (1953). The effect of the structure of the ego on psychoanalytic technique. *Journal of the American Psychoanalytic Association*. 1:104-143.

———. (1958). Notes on problems of technique in the psychoanalytic treatment of adolescents: with some remarks on perversion. *Psychoanalytic Study of the Child*. 13:223-254.

Geleerd, Elisabeth R. (1967). Ed. *The Child Analyst at Work*. 1-13. New York: International Universities Press.

Harley, Marjorie (1961). Some observations on the relationship between genitality and structural development at adolescence. *Journal of the American Psychoanalytic Association*. 9:434-460.

————. (1971). Some reflections on identity problems in prepuberty. In: *Separation-individuation* 385-403. New York: International Universities Press.

Hartmann, Heinz (1951). Technical implications of ego psychology. In: *Essays on Ego Psychology*. 142-154. New York: International Universities Press.

The Analyst and the Adolescent at Work

The Technique of Defense Analysis in the Psychoanalysis of an Early Adolescent

Calvin F. Settlage, M.D.   *San Francisco*

INTRODUCTION

Geleerd (1957) and Eissler (1958) underscored what has proved to be a continuing concern among psychoanalysts with the application of the analytic method to adolescents. These authors were among the first to observe that the clarifications and modifications of psychoanalytic technique which resulted from advances in the psychoanalytic understanding of the ego (Freud, 1923; Anna Freud, 1936; and Hartmann, 1939) were particularly pertinent to adolescent analysis.

Geleerd (1957) noted that a special effort has to be made in adolescent analysis to increase the tolerance of the ego to pathogenic conflicts. At the same time, she cautioned that the analysis of defenses in adolescence harbors the danger of surrendering the adolescent to his id. Eissler (1958) called attention to the process of reorganization which is normally part of adolescent development and stressed the need for flexibility in technique. He felt that the great changeability in the dynamics of adolescent functioning and in symptoms, not only from day to day but from minute to minute in a given analytic session, means that no one technique can fulfill the requirements for the treatment of adolescents.

More recently, Maenchen (1970), also emphasizing the con-

3

tribution of ego psychology, observes that the overemphasis of any one approach to unconscious material leads to a one-sided and possibly a lopsided view of analytic material. Of the several perspectives one might choose in attempting to gain a fresh view on problems of technique, namely, symptomatology, transference, superego or ego functions, she finds that of ego functions to be the most promising. To paraphrase her, not only are the ego functions readily accessible to observation in analysis, but the relative immaturity or inadequacy of the patient's ego enters into the determination of the details of analytic technique. The latter is the case whether the immaturity or inadequacy is due to development still being in process, as in the child or adolescent, or due to neurotically determined defensive impairment of ego functions. Maenchen notes that the state of flux in the adolescent personality, conveyed by Eissler's (1958) reference to the process of reorganization in this phase, was at one time used as a reason against adolescent analysis, but is now given as a reason for it.[1] Maenchen's viewpoint is summarized in her statement:

- Technique, then, is dictated not by symptomatology alone or the developmental stage, but by the actual and particular state of ego functioning in its connection with psychopathology. One could say that it is this causal relation between the state of ego functions and the symptomatology which dictates technique (p. 185).

Because of the developmental immaturity of the child, child analysts have had to address themselves to the question of differences between technical adaptations compatible with the analytic method and incompatible technical deviations. Marianne Kris (Casuso, 1965) proposed that the term *adaptations* be used for modifications in technique required by the developmental level of the child and by the need to create an analytic therapeutic climate.

Maenchen (1970) also discusses the difference between adaptation of analytic technique in keeping with the child's level of development and the use of technical parameters. She offers the following clarifying statement, which she credits to Philip M. Spielman.

- [The term] "parameter" should be used to designate deviations in technique necessitated by the patient's psychopathology (ego strength, nature of anxiety, extent of regression), and "adaptations" should be reserved for modifications in the approach appropriate to different developmental levels (with no pathology implied) and to technical shifts in relation to new developmental phases in the same patient. . . . both terms should be distinguished from "errors in technique" which are based on the analyst's incorrect assessment of the child and his needs (p. 197).

In my view, there is a distinct value, more clearly evident in analyzing children but no less important in analyzing adolescents and adults, in distinguishing between adaptations and other modifications of technique. A technical adaptation is employed when an analytically necessary ego function is lacking because of the position of the child in the continuum of normal development or because of neurotically determined, defensive impairment. A technical deviation is employed because the basic elements of the analytic situation cannot at the time be met, or because the patient's ego capacities and functions are seriously impaired by more severe psychopathology. As thus defined, adaptations of technique do not compromise the basic principles and aims of the analytic method, whereas parametric modifications or deviations do.

Although he was addressing himself to the technique of adult analysis, rather than child or adolescent analysis, Loewenstein's (1967) views are pertinent to the preceding discussion. He expressed himself as follows:

- The psychoanalyst uses essentially his patient's autonomous functions to initiate and further the analytic process, and to assist in leading to a satisfactory result. Even in order to follow the fundamental rule, the patient must have at his disposal a number of complex autonomous ego functions such as anticipation, reality testing in a wide sense, speech, self-observation, as well as relatively stable object relations. And those of his functions which are in any way inhibited or disturbed by resistance—that is, in some part by the defence[2]—must be assisted by the activities of the analyst. It is correct to say, I believe, that in this respect the analyst has the function of a temporary, auxiliary autonomous ego for his patient (p. 800).

(See also Loewenstein, 1954, 1956.)

In keeping with the views of Maenchen and child analysts generally, Loewenstein (1967) goes on to say:

- We must distinguish between two sides of the psychoanalytic technique: on the one hand, the method and procedures and specific technical rules; on the other hand, the use of analytic knowledge in order to implement this method, so that the analytic process can unfold and lead to a satisfactory termination (pp. 800-801).

In commenting upon the above presented views, I wish to stress first that all of the authors are, at least as I understand them, calling attention to and suggesting the need for adaptations in standard analytic technique (as developed originally in treating neurotic adults) *with the aim of being able to fulfill the purposes of the analytic method*. Second, I subscribe to the view that psychoanalytic ego psychology provides the basis for such adaptations of technique. Third, I feel that the technique of defense analysis, as it has continued to evolve, provides a sound approach to the analysis of children and adolescents and is one which challenges Eissler's (1956) view that no one technique can fulfill the requirements for the treatment of adolescents. In my experience, this technique of defense analysis also answers Geleerd's (1957) concern about surrendering the adolescent to his id, and Bornstein's (1949) caution against pushing the ego beyond its integrative powers. Further, it is my impression that defense analysis has for many analysts become an integral part of standard technique in the analysis of adults.

THE CONCEPT AND TECHNIQUE
OF DEFENSE ANALYSIS

It is my impression that *defense analysis* means quite different things to different analysts. Accordingly, I shall set forth what it means to me, at the same time reviewing, pulling together, and commenting upon contributions to the literature on this subject.[3]

Perhaps *the central tenet of defense analysis is the recognition that the position of the ego and its need for defense is to be respected*. Put in the broadest terms, this tenet is reflected in Greenson's observations (Pumpian-Mindlin, 1967, p. 155) that "the analyst's ultimate aim is to enable the patient's ego to cope better with the id, the superego, and the external world." What underlies this principle is an acceptance of the following facts: that the patient's presenting symptoms and defenses represent his current best compromise solution to the unconscious conflicts; that the unconscious conflicts, repressed during earlier development, have remained unchanged and the possibility of their emergence into conscious awareness continues to engender anxiety despite the patient's now older, further developed, and generally more capable ego; and that a too direct or too rapid attempt at exposure of warded-off material tends, therefore, to provoke a hardening of the defenses and resistances and pose a threat to the therapeutic alliance. Because of the successive increments of insight and mastery over warded-off material which defense analysis gradually provides, the ego is strengthened increasingly as the analysis proceeds and its position viv-à-vis the id or the superego is similarly improved. Weiss (1971) stresses that it is a strengthening of the patient's ego which enables the emergence of previously warded-off content, and discusses the circumstances which may lead to such a strengthening.

Strengthening and improving the position of the ego is particularly valuable in the analysis of a patient whose ego is greatly threatened by, and tightly defending against, his instinctual forces. As has been well elucidated (A. Freud, 1936, 1958; GAP6, 1968), the early adolescent is characteristically a prime example of such a patient. In addition to the internal disruption caused by psychopathology, the changes initiated by puberty make this threatened position of the ego the usual and normal condition during early adolescence.

A *second tenet of defense analysis holds that analysis of the defense and what it defends against are to be pursued simultaneously.* Analysis of a defense is not undertaken in isolation from the reasons for it, or without considering the question of its role in the overall balance of intrapsychic forces. A judgment as to the appropriateness of approaching a particular defense at a particular time is made in the context of an understanding of the patient's total defensive and adaptive stance.[4] The technique may involve the temporary allowance of certain defensive avoidances or even the strengthening of certain defenses, because the impulse-defense configuration suggests that it is, at that time, wise to do so. Defense analysis, then, is simultaneously concerned with both the defense and the drive aspect of the patient's behavior.

Fenichel (1941) was quite specific about this: "By no means is a given phenomenon always *either* defense and in the ego *or* instinct and in the id. *Derivatives* always compromise *both*" (p. 57). Gill (1963) speaks of impulse-defense units, and Waelder (Pumpian-Mindlin, 1967) states that "challenges of the id and responses of the ego should be analyzed together" (p. 152).

Gill (1963) noted that the steps in the technique of defense analysis are: (1) to make clear to the patient *that* he wards off something; (2) *how* he does it; (3) *what* he is warding off (as enunciated by Reich, 1933); and (4) *why* he does it (as added by Fenichel, 1945). The defense, as expressed in the patient's observable behavior can, as a rule, be more readily inferred by the analyst and more readily faced and acknowledged by the patient than can the associated unconscious impulse or conflict. The analytic sequence usually proceeds, therefore, from observation of verbal or nonverbal behavior, to inference of defense, to the discovery of the reasons for the defense. The question of why the defense is needed is, however, presented to the patient simultaneously with the delineation of the defense, thus directing his attention toward the unknown which lies immediately ahead, and inviting his participation in the searching and uncovering process. In defense analysis, dynamic interpretation—that is, of the forces determining the patient's current behavior in the analytic situation—tends to precede and set the stage for transference interpretation and genetic interpretation of the correlated infantile determinants.

Important to the rationale of defense analysis is the concept of layering of defenses. The key elements in this concept are that there is a hierarchical arrangement of defenses, and that, in this stratification, certain defenses and what they defend against are nearer and less threatening to conscious perception than others. *In the technique of defense analysis, attention is focused on these most superficial layers of defense, on the basis that the ego will have a greater tolerance for exposure of warded-off contents at this level than at deeper and more tightly defended levels.* As a particular defense and the immediately underlying unconscious material which it has been defending are interpreted and dealt with, the next and somewhat deeper layer comes into view. Thus the process tends to proceed stepwise from the more superficial toward the deeper levels of unconscious material, and in the progression from superficial to deeper levels, earlier and more primitive defenses tend to be encountered.[5]

As has been noted by Gill (1953), characterization of the process of defense analysis makes both the process and the layering of the psychic apparatus sound unrealistically orderly and mechanistic. In practice, the process does not proceed smoothly from layer to layer, nor does it deal first with one psychopathological theme and then another. Rather, it moves back and forth from layer to layer, and from theme to theme, as the patient's presenting defenses shift in response to the changing anxieties engendered by the analysis and by the vicissitudes of the patient's daily life situation. Nevertheless, the direction and form of the process is as described, and the related technical principle holds—that is, to meet the patient wherever he is in his current defensive postures and to tackle first those defenses and that defended content which one judges to be least threatening to the ego.

In regard to a perhaps still controversial point, *defense analysis does not remove or destroy the defenses; nor does it force the patient to yield his defenses.* The use of defenses is an essential part of normal ego function and adaptation. Rather, in conjunction with working through, defense analysis tends to remove the pathologic need for the defense in relation to the specific unconscious issue being dealt with at that particular point in the course of the analysis. Ernst Kris (Zetzel, 1954) expressed a similar understanding:

- Successful analysis will not result in the abolition of defenses, but rather in their modification and increased appropriateness. [He suggested] that three changes are of decisive importance: (1) the diminution of instinctual danger will diminish the need for pathogenic defenses; (2) the analysis of ego fixations will have increased —though to a limited degree—the number of available defenses; and (3) the appropriate operation of the modified defenses and the associated release of neutralized instinctual energy will inevitably lead to increased autonomous ego function (p. 321).

THE PSYCHOANALYSIS OF AN EARLY ADOLESCENT

Having reviewed, discussed, and defined the concept and technique of defense analysis in broad terms, I now aim to demonstrate its application in, and its particular suitability for, the analysis of the early adolescent. In attempting to so demonstrate, I will present examples of the technique used, along with sufficient reasons for these and sufficient evidence of their influence on the patient, to convey the analytic process. While the excerpts which I have selected may also convey some impression of the patient's progress, I am not endeavoring to give a comprehensive picture of the analysis.

After formulation of the clinical problem, my approach will be to state first what I regard as the generic principle of defense analysis and then to show how it can be implemented. The more specific principles which I shall illustrate are: steadfast alliance with the patient's ego; temporarily allowing and even facilitating distancing of the ego from too threatening, warded-off material; tentatively mapping out the unknown territory of the unconscious mind suspected to lie immediately ahead; and improving the position of the ego by giving the patient understanding of his psychic processes and their purposes.

THE CLINICAL PROBLEM

Harry, age 14, was the youngest of two children in a closely knit, upper-middle-class family. His sibling was a girl three years his senior. The father was a college professor and the mother a college educated housewife with many interests and activities. The family had a liberal social and political outlook and placed a high value on intellectual achievement and the arts.

Harry came to treatment primarily because of his concern about his symptom of ''mind freezing.'' At certain times, he would be temporarily unable to continue his activities, such as doing his homework, because of a thought about someone from his current or past life whom he regarded as intellectually and culturally inferior to himself and his family. He had the fear that whatever he was thinking and learning at the time, always valued knowledge, ''would be lost and go to that person.'' Frequently, there was the simultaneous juxtaposition of the negatively regarded person to someone whom he regarded very highly, with a fantasied fusion of their images which carried the threat of ''loss'' of the valued person. He dealt with these fears by a compulsive, stepwise retracing in his mind of all of the valued thoughts surrounding the onset of the symptom. If he carried out this laborious and time-consuming process in precisely the right way, he could regain his lost knowledge and undo the fusion, thus achieving restitution. The symptoms had become so frequent, occurring many times a day, that they were interfering with Harry's generally outstanding school performance, and were changing his normally congenial, very alive disposition into one of tension, constriction, and remoteness.

Physically, Harry was well into puberty. Yet, his slender, rather delicate build, his physical demeanor, and his general manner, which included an excess of politeness and agreeability, gave the impression that he was more in latency than early adolescence. As the analysis proceeded, the reason for his demeanor and manner became evident. Harry revealed that, despite his awareness of changes due to puberty, it was his fervent wish to remain a little boy, to ward off adolescence. He resented the inevitability of his physical growth which was now threatening to make him taller than anyone in the family. He also wanted to preserve the intactness of the family, freezing it in time as it were, and thus perpetuating his position and his adaptation as the youngest child. Contained within his wish not to grow up was the fear of growing old, of death and dying.

Historically, death and loss were a significant part of Harry's childhood years, both actual loss and libidinal loss[6] or the threat of it. The actual losses, all of which appeared to have been emotionally significant, included the following: at age 8, the death of his paternal grandmother, and, at 9, of his paternal grandfather, with both of whom he had been very close; at age 10, the moving away of a best friend as a result of this friend's parents' divorce; at age 11, the suicide of a close friend's mother; at age 12 and a half, the moving away of another friend after the friend's house had burned down; at age 13, shortly after Harry's return from what for him had been a very important trip to South America, the sudden death of his dog. Following the death of the grandparents, his earlier fear of death became a steady concern. To illustrate the intensity of this concern, when Harry's mother discarded some house plants which were quite obviously dead, he retrieved them and watered them for several weeks, hoping to revive them.

While the actual losses occurred psychogenetically quite late during development, the libidinal losses or threats of loss, which became clear only through reconstruction in the analysis, were experienced during early childhood. The reconstruction began with numbers of similar current experiences involving Harry and his mother. Typically, his mother responded with anger and much exaggerated objections to any of Harry's moves toward autonomy and independence for which she was unprepared. For example, Harry, now a 15-year-old, called her one day after school to say that he would not be home for dinner. He had forgotten to tell her that morning about a late afternoon class outing. His mother became very upset and angry, objected on the grounds that she was expecting him for dinner, and complained that she had prepared it for nought—all of this despite the fact that the rest of the family would be at home for dinner. On his part, Harry responded to such episodes with feelings of guilt and contrition, and renewed strivings to please his mother so as to remain close to her.

Harry's recollections from early childhood included many admonitions from his mother about the dangers in the neighborhood while, at the same time, she encouraged him to be independent and permitted him to play away from home. During these years, too, she seemingly became unduly upset and angry when he tarried longer than expected. While Harry's mother was in fact knowledgeable, conscientious, and devoted in her mothering, and while she consciously encouraged the development of autonomy and independence in her children, it appeared that her own unresolved neurotic conflicts caused an overanxious, unreasonable reaction to unexpected, disturbing events and situations wherein she felt loss of control.

One can postulate that this circumstance caused Harry's developmental separation experiences and moves toward independence to be surrounded by an aura of danger, and that the threat of loss of love implicit in his mother's anger fostered an underaggressive, conforming attachment to her. In short, the separation-individuation process, formulated by Mahler (1965, 1968) failed to reach an adequate resolution in Harry, primarily because of his defensive blocking of the expression and modulation of sexual and aggressive urges and affects. Aggression was essentially denied and gained its only expression in highly disguised form, as, for example, in the initially unrecognized competitiveness in the area of intellectual prowess and acquisition of knowledge. During the previously mentioned important trip to South America, Harry's latent interest in Latin American cultures had blossomed into an intense preoccupation. As an illustration of the veiled expression of aggression, he fantasied that he would come to know more about ancient Latin American cultures than anyone in history, and would, through his writings and renown, live forever in the halls of academia. While sexuality was expressed more overtly, it was on an intellectual fantasy level, and the sexual feelings normally associated with such fantasy were significant by their absence. For example, during the analysis Harry revealed that he was currently playing a ''game'' with his sister in which he was the chronically rejected suitor for her hand in marriage. He was unaware of any sexual feelings during the game despite the fact that it included close physical contact; and he unanxiously acknowledged the incestuous nature of the fantasies, seemingly feeling protected by his defensive posture of being and remaining a little boy. Early in the treatment he had none of the typical, early adolescent's professed interest in girls.

The patient's fear of loss of impulse control—the other side of his tightly controlled, conforming behavior—was first revealed in his dreams. In his first reported dream, the patient was on the moon where a man, who was in charge of a processing machine, removed his own head and placed it in the machine. The machine was supposed to change it, hopefully but not clearly for the good, and then return it. This dream came to be understood as representing the patient's defensive separation of mind from body, of the rational refined intellect from the irrational, crude, animalistic passions. Occurring at the beginning of treatment, it also expressed the patient's anticipatory fear of what the analyst and the analytical process might do to him. The analyst would tamper with his delicately balanced mind-body dichotomy. In unraveling his symptom and helping him ''grow up,'' the analysis would separate him from his mother and his family both psychologically and physically (symbolically, sending him to the moon), thus depriving him of the external support upon which he so much relied for control of his urges.

In another dream, early in the analysis, the patient was standing on the edge of a precipice, fearing that he might jump off into space. As he explicated in discussing the dream, he was afraid that his body would act on the thought of jumping before his mind could tell it not to jump. The fear of urges and impulses was, to my mind, the inevitable corollary of the patient's general, defensive style.

What can be inferred from both these dreams is that the patient managed a not very substantial ego control over an instinctual life that had been dealt with mainly by denial and exclusion, and as something alien, unwanted, to be disavowed. Such an internal state—in Maenchen's (1970) terms, the state of ego functioning in its connection with psychopathology—requires particular emphasis on the analytic technique of defense analysis. As I understood the patient's predicament and psychopathology, the thrust of puberty was renewing the fears and anxieties first associated with his unresolved infantile separation-individuation and later perpetuated in an equally unresolved oedipal conflict; and the defensive and adaptive measures which he forged at those earlier times were now being challenged by the pressure toward independent adult functioning which is such a central factor in adolescence. Because of the unresolved, earlier developmental issues, the patient was ill prepared to confront the second *individuation* of adolescence (Blos, 1967).[7]

PRINCIPLES AND TECHNIQUES

The earlier stated tenet of *alliance with the patient's ego* with the aim of strengthening it and gradually improving its ability to cope with the id, the superego, and the external world is, to my mind, the generic principle of defense analysis, inherent also in the more specific analytic principles and techniques. This principle is illustrated by the nature of the transference in the beginning of Harry's analysis. While transference attitudes and expectations were evident in the material, they were not at all overt, and the patient consistently shunned recognizing or talking about his thoughts and feelings concerning the analyst.

In an hour several months into the analysis, the patient associatively exposed some of his previously carefully guarded anxieties and fantasies regarding his aggressive urges. The stimulus for the hour was an automobile crash which he had witnessed. He recalled the time, during latency, when he had crashed his bike into that of another boy and then had been teased and poked by the boy and his friends. He then remembered another time when he had engaged in rough-and-tumble play with several of his peers and had ended up the last one on "another guy's back." The guy had said, "What's this flea doing on my back?" The patient had been humiliated and angry. The next association was to the time when his paternal uncle had been bitten by an insect, a bad bite which had made his uncle very sick and which had required medical treatment. Later in the same hour, he mentioned an incident on a family vacation trip. His father had held him by the legs so he could safely look down into a deep, seemingly bottomless, old well. At the time he had been very frightened, thinking that his father's grasp might slip, and he later had a scary dream of walking through fields full of dangerous holes and pits. When asked whether he could see any significance in the sequence of his thoughts, the patient was able to recognize the theme of aggressive behavior being followed by a bad consequence. He crashed into another guy and got teased and poked; symbolically, he, the insignificant but angry flea, bit and inflicted serious damage but was then in danger of falling into pits or bottomless holes.

The patient failed to show up for the next appointment. He said it had "just slipped his mind." When he next came, he reported a dream from the night before the missed appointment. In the dream, he was vigorously disagreeing and arguing with his mother, something new to his dreams and something feared and avoided in his waking life. The patient did not at first connect the dream with the fact that his mother had voiced, during the day preceding the dream, her strong disapproval of one of the patient's friends because the friend was not sufficiently polite. When the patient recalled the content of the previous hour and connected it with the dream of arguing with his mother, I interpreted to him that he had forgotten the appointment because he feared I was going to get him into trouble by exposing and stirring up his aggressive urges and feelings. Whereas I might have sought the patient's associations to the oedipal implications of the material in the hour before the missed appointment, I chose not to do so in either of these sessions. I felt that both the general tenor of the material, and his response to my much less specific inquiry about the possible significance of the sequence of his thoughts, indicated the terms in which his ego could safely approach the material.

Some months later, the same kind of fear surfaced in relation to sexual urges. The patient began an hour with a gratuitous reaffirmation of his repeatedly declared interest in the pursuit of knowledge toward his chosen career in archeology. Recalling an earlier noted concern that he was now sometimes neglecting his studies in favor of having fun, he mentioned that he would never become like the Beach Boys, the rock 'n' roll recording group which he felt was dedicated solely to the pursuit of pleasure. He then volunteered a dream which had the following sequences: he was in a small room with white walls, which contained the detached head of a statue; he was riding on a bus which went past the analyst's office on its way downtown; and, he was shopping in a Mexican market where he objected to the Mexicans' use of Americanized "Madison Avenue" sales techniques. The small room with the white walls reminded him of the analyst's office, and he recalled that he had recently thought about how he and the analyst were closed within the office; it made him feel uneasy. In connection with "white" he said he had recently read that white stands for death in the Asian culture. He had also been reading about hara-kiri. As an afterthought, he wondered whether the detached head could be connected with the much earlier reported dream about the man who took off his own head and put it into the machine which was supposed to change it. Significantly, it was in the preceding hour that the patient had first revealed that he played the earlier mentioned sex game with his sister. In line with the principle of alliance with the ego, I chose not to press, at this time, for the patient's further associations to the subjects of death, hara-kiri (self-destruction), or the sex game. Instead, I told him that he seemed again to be expressing his fear that I, with my analytic techniques, was causing him to change, and undesirably so, this time by beginning to unleash his sexual feelings and urges.

Such fears are, at least in some measure, a part of every analysis, but they are crucially intense in the early adolescent. As I have previously noted, the neurotically repressed and denied needs, urges, and affects, reengendered by the analytic situation and experienced in the transference, compound the internal threat to the ego from the normal, developmentally determined surge of the instinctual drives. The patient reacts fearfully, therefore, to the analyst's seeming encouragement of the instinctual forces.

The just presented illustrations are, I believe, in keeping with Weiss's (1971) stress on the patient's need to feel safe with the analyst in order to expose warded-off material. Weiss emphasizes the neutrality and nonreactiveness of the analyst as the basis for this feeling of safety. As another basis, I would add the analyst's alliance with and working through the ego, as determined by his cumulative understanding of the patient's psychopathology and psychodynamics, his estimate of the current balance of intra-psychic forces in the specific analytic hour, and his best judgment as to the probable impact at this point in time of a possible line of inquiry or specific interpretive intervention, otherwise tenable on the basis of the content of the hour, per se.

A second principle of defense analysis is what has been referred to as *distancing*.[8] As I would formulate it, this concept holds that the defensively maintained distance between the conscious, rational ego and the unconscious, warded-off mental contents should be closed at a pace and in a manner tolerable to the ego. Distancing stresses the importance of ego preparation, of timing, of control, and of mastery through putting psychic experiences into words.

Loewenstein (1956), noting how a patient's words had carried a previously unconscious thought and affect to the surface of conscious awareness, suggested that language performs the function of a kind of scaffolding that permits conscious thought to be built inside. He added that the same might be said of the analyst's interpretations which provide another scaffolding which the patient's thought can *gradually* fill (my italics). Weiss (1971), speaking specifically of defense analysis, elaborates on the means by which word symbols can lead to increased ego control.

In reviewing the analysis of this verbal, intellectual, scholarly young adolescent, it strikes me that the only possible analytic approach was, at least for a long time, to allow him his intellectual-verbal defense, and even capitalize upon it, as a means of supporting ego control over the threatening urges and affects, analyzing it at a later, more favorable time. While this defense, which is certainly in the direction of intellectualization, is commonly used as a resistance and its facilitation by the analyst is normally to be guarded against, the situation in Harry's case was quite different. This is well illustrated by the patient's completely unsolicited and persistent use of his dream as the primary basis for communication, particularly in the first part of the analysis. For a time I was indeed concerned that this represented a resistance, an impediment to the analytic work, but the concern seemed unwarranted in the face of the fact that the analysis was progressing in a satisfactory way.

My understanding of my patient's use of his dreams is in accord with concepts enunciated by Harley (1962). In the analysis of a latency-age girl heavily burdened by the pressures of her inner urgencies, Harley noted that the dream provided both a "safety valve" for the discharge of the patient's excessive excitations and a means of substituting reflective thought for impulsive action. The dream thus enabled Harley's patient to achieve distance from her unconscious material, not to escape it but to view and approach it without the fear of being overwhelmed by it.

What Harley formulated about the use of dreams by the latency-age child is equally valid for the adolescent: analytic technique should respect the patient's endeavors to meet the maturational demands for supremacy of the secondary process, and help him to circumvent the primary-process threat of the dream. This formulation does not negate the long-standing dictum that the dream is "the royal road to the unconscious," but it does suggest that the road be traveled with care and certainly not in haste.

The need for distancing as a means of respecting the maturational demand for supremacy of the secondary process during early adolescence is illustrated by the earlier presented formulation of the defensive mind-body dichotomization expressed in the dreams containing references to detached heads. An illustration of this technique from an early point in the analysis begins with Harry's reporting a dream which was replete with rushing, spurting waters, in streams, waterfalls, and tunnels. In one part of the dream, his father was standing on a footbridge suspended over a rushing stream which ended in a towering waterfall. In contrast to the activity and tension in the dream, Harry told it in a very casual, matter-of-fact way. Because the latter defensive attitudes suggested a need for distancing, I elected not to pick up on the phallic, oedipal, competitive implications of the dream. I decided instead to call attention to two details which I suspected of having anal implications: the fact that the tunnel system was open at one point so that he could look down on a whirlpool of rushing, swirling, noisy waters; and that the tunnels would change direction and shunt the water, for example, at a right angle to its previous course, as if it were in a water pipe.

Harry's associations indeed led him to the idea of water in pipes and to his childhood curiosity about what happened to the water flushed down the toilet. He recalled having once worried about an insect in the toilet bowl and how it would feel going through the pipes. He then had a seemingly unrelated recollection from age 6 of standing on a cliff next to the beginning of a waterfall and fearing that he would fall into the water and be carried over the brink, even though his father was holding him by the hand. This caused him to remember an early childhood fear of falling into the toilet. He also recalled thinking that he was losing something of himself in his bowel movement. He next revealed, in connection with his symptom, that he had in the past been afraid his knowledge could be lost in his feces. Finally, he mentioned that he sometimes concretizes the notion of losing knowledge from his head, visualizing his thoughts as a tangible, solid mass and making restitutive gestures of poking a chunk of knowledge back into his head.

This material is cited primarily to illustrate how the patient used his dream as a distancing device and how this need was respected in the analytic technique. At the same time, it is noteworthy that this technique proved to be analytically fruitful. The dream and the thus garnered associations to it indicate developmental linkages between fear of loss in connection with having a bowel movement and castration fear (Settlage, 1971), as well as between these and the fear of death, and the upwardly displaced fear, during adolescence, of loss of knowledge. The rather cautious technical approach, which might be regarded as unnecessarily circuitous, not only was not exploited by the patient for the purposes of resistance but led to his bringing forth new, psychologically deep and genetically early material which moved him closer to, rather than farther away from, his castration anxiety.

This same material also illustrates distancing by dealing with issues first in terms of the more distant past rather than the more recent past, the anal phase before the oedipal or adolescent phases. This distancing measure may be spontaneous on the patient's part or can, as in this instance, be used deliberately as a part of the analytic technique. *When the analyst feels that the patient cannot as yet deal with currently stirred-up but threatening, warded-off material*, in some instances, it may be helpful to inquire quite directly as to whether the material suggests any experiences or remembrances from earlier childhood. Parenthetically, the natural tendency of the associative process to go in the direction of childhood may be determined in part by the need for distancing.

Another technique which provides both distancing and ego preparation is that of broadening the field. The threat of overtly or latently, affectively highly charged material, and the consequent strengthening of resistances, can sometimes be moderated by directing the patient's attention to contiguous but less intense areas, through comments or questions. As an example, Harry was, in a particular hour, becoming increasingly discouraged, distraught, and upset with himself as he talked of his inability to prevent the intrusion of his symptom into his studies. He noted this was especially difficult whenever he was nearing the end of a given segment of work. When asked about the latter observation, the patient revealed that upon finishing his studies he literally jumped or fled into bed, not permitting himself to sit and think or relax for a while and sometimes not even brushing his teeth. This revelation appeared both to add to the patient's distress and concomitantly to increase his resistances. *In order to relieve the pressure of the moment*, the technique of broadening the field was employed. The patient's attention was deliberately directed away from his obsessive preoccupation with his learning difficulties by asking him whether he had had trouble with bedtime or sleep during his childhood.

Harry then had a series of recollections having to do with beds, bedtime, and sleep in earlier years, and as he spoke of them his tension, distress, and attitude of self-depreciation subsided. The patient remembered that his first "big" bed was provided by his now deceased paternal grandfather. He wanted it but feared he might fall out of it. At age 7 or 8, he used to hide under the covers for fear of a witch who he fantasied would come in the middle of the night and take him away to a hidden cave where his parents would never find him. He imagined how he would appease the witch with a trinity of thoughts: "I like you; people who think ill of you are wrong; I'll be on your side when you steal from the grocery store and are chased." At age 5 or 6 he routinely jumped into bed from several feet away in order to avoid having his ankles clutched by dangerous humanoid creatures that he imagined to be lurking under the bed.

The material thus brought out was again most relevant to the understanding of the patient's problem, and provided preparation for the later exposure of the oedipal fantasies and fear of castration, connected as they were with his fear of death, of *ending*. At the same time, the technique of broadening the field averted the impasse and potential resistance which were developing because of the patient's inability to deal, at this point in the analysis, with the affects being stirred up around these issues.

A third principle of defense analysis, of particular value in the analysis of the early adolescent, is the *tentative mapping out of the unknown territory of the unconscious mind suspected to lie immediately ahead*. From the viewpoint of the patient's ego, knowing and being able to anticipate what is likely to come reduce the threat of being totally surprised and overwhelmed.

An example in Harry's case stemmed from the following sequence, the elements of which were, to him, at first unconnected. He spoke at length about the movie *L'Enfant Sauvage*, stressing only how enjoyable it was; he talked next about his fear of making people angry; and he then deplored the persistence of his symptom, his fear of losing knowledge to others and having ritualistically to regain it. When his own associations shed no light on why this sequence of topics, I pointed out that there seemed to be a rather obvious progression from talk about the savage, uncontrolled infant, to awareness of his fear that he might do something to make people angry, to thoughts about his symptom. I reminded him of our earlier discussion of how it appeared that his own childhood experiences caused him to wish to separate his mind from his body as a means of escaping and controlling urges and feelings which seemed to threaten particularly his relationship with his mother. I then stated that I would expect his long-standing worry about loss of control to be aggravated because of his now being an adolescent, since fear of one's impulses is normally a problem in adolescence. One of the areas which he was probably unconsciously avoiding but which we would be looking at was that of his adolescent sexual and aggressive fantasies and feelings.

Harry began the following hour with a discussion of the beauty and purity of some ancient South American artifacts which he had recently seen in a local museum. He spoke also of his feeling of excitement and of an impending climax as he listened to a university professor lecture. He then revealed that he was planning to go to the university library to look up some books reputed to have some "dirty, sexy" pictures about certain Aztec ceremonial functions. Here he harked back to the previous analytic session and said he guessed he was interested in sex, and he realized that thinking about sexy pictures did stir up sexual feelings. Because of my impression that Harry could only slowly expose his sexual fantasies and activities, for the time being I intentionally ignored the quite evident representation of a masturbatory equivalent with orgasm which was expressed in relation to the lecture. I felt that his acknowledgment of having sexual curiosity and feelings was quite enough as a first step.

Another example of the mapping out of the unknown began with Harry's report of having read an article in which a number of outstanding professors represented statements on the present and future directions of the fields of history, philosophy, and biology. He first stated that he was, surprisingly to him, getting interested in biology, a subject he had always derogated. His next comment was, however, a put-down of biology: "The field is dull and no good. It changes terribly slowly, maybe a little bit over a twenty-to-thirty-year period."

When it was shortly clear that he had dropped the subject, I brought Harry back to it, pointing out his quick disavowal of his new interest in biology. I suggested that this interest might reflect a wish to learn about and come to terms with his own adolescent biological self, but that he was at the same time fearful of what he might discover. After a moment's reflection he said that he thought this was so. He then volunteered the seeming digression that he had noticed he was of late beginning to look at the bad side of the ancient South American cultures. Heretofore he had only idealized and aggrandized them. He was puzzled and a bit worried by this, fearing it might mean he was *losing* his determined dedication to his chosen career.

Harry's attention was again directed to the unknown in himself, this time in terms of his needing and wanting to acknowledge and deal with what he felt to be the bad part of himself, something he had always consciously disavowed. The need to divorce his mind from his body was again mentioned, now with the aim of opening the door to the subject of how he had apparently tried to deal with good and bad, both outside and inside himself, by splitting them and keeping them apart. From previous discussions, he was aware that he tended to classify people as either all good or all bad. I shared with him my hunch that his striving toward becoming the brilliant, renowned professor of archeology at the expense of having no time for fun—his need to become the perfect, ascetic "compleat" man—was a compensation for a somewhere felt, but denied, bad deficient self.[9]

In the next hour Harry reported a dream in which the father of a guy whom he disliked had poked Harry in the back "with a nail or something. It really hurt." Harry had no particular thoughts about the dream but, when asked what the poking in the back brought to mind, he mentioned that his mother poked him in the back to make him sit up straight, doing it even in front of company. He chuckled as he gave this information, at first denying that it bothered him, but later acknowledging that it did make him feel a twinge of anger.

Harry then recalled reading about two tribes in northern New Guinea who lived on opposite sides of a big hill, although he did not know why this came to mind. They were constantly at war with each other, much of the time in sham, gestural warfare, but sometimes in fierce mortal combat. Intriguingly, whenever a child died in either tribe, the tribes would get together in a harmonious feast of sadness and mourning which yielded to happiness and even elation. After this temporary peace, the age-old hostilities would again be resumed. This associative material can be suspected of having many implications, but it was used at this time as the basis for interpreting to Harry that he was afraid the analyst's "nudgings or pokings" would stir up his anger and aggression and get him into conflict with the analyst, and that this transference fear had its roots in his childhood relationship with his mother. Rather than dealing with the transference at this time, I went on to observe that his recollection, just now, of the warring tribes which also came together in peace suggested that he wanted to reconcile not only the conflicts of the present and past between himself and his mother, but the conflicting and split-apart, good-bad elements in himself. I explained that it was likely these conflicting elements had resulted from his understandable need, during early childhood, to please his mother and retain her love, doing so by submerging his angry, aggressive, bad feelings and urges. Further, I pointed out that the part of his symptom which tended to fuse a good person with a bad person seemed to be a reflection of this same desire for reconciliation and internal harmony.

A fourth principle of defense analysis is *improvement of the position of the ego by giving the patient understanding of his psychic processes and their purposes*. This principle is validly applied only in relation to specific analytic material and only when it can be of value to the patient in understanding and dealing with factors in the current balance of inner forces. It is not to be construed as a sanction for "educating" the patient about mental mechanisms or other concepts in isolation from dynamically meaningful analytic material, a practice which would serve no other purpose than the undesirable one of playing into the hands of resistance.

The above discussion with Harry of the defense of splitting and why he needed it in his early childhood, and of the probable derivation and purpose of his perfectionistic strivings are examples of the application of this principle. Another example arose from exploration of the patient's fear of forgetting as being due to causes within himself, whereas the fear of losing knowledge to others he attributed to inexplicable, outside forces. It was explained to the patient that his fear of forgetting could be based on the fact that he wanted to "forget" or repress certain things which he regarded as alien to himself, and which, if remembered, would stir up troublesome feelings. The problem was that this forgetting, since it was not consciously directed, might also include things which he did not want to forget. Noting the similarity between the new fear of forgetting and the old symptom of fearing his knowledge would be lost to others, I reminded him that he had come to know that there was a part of himself which he wanted to deny, namely, his competitive, aggressive, bad, and perhaps even destructive self. It seemed that he had in the past tried to escape this part of himself by externalizing it as the mysterious force which could make him lose his knowledge to others, and which he fought against in the restitutive aspect of his symptom.[10]

The patient responded with the confirming illustration of his lack of fear of forgetting when he was in the classroom situation. He realized that he told himself that he was there just for the sake of learning itself and, while there, he never imagined using the acquired knowledge to compete in the future and become a famous man who would go down in the pages of history. Hence, by this process of intellectualization, he kept both the fear and the symptom from occurring in the classroom. Pertinently, Harry reported in a later hour that the understanding gained from my explanations had helped him deal with the symptom while studying at home.

Another example had to do with Harry's residual fantasies of omnipotence. These emerged in his admiring but anxiously ambivalent discussion of kings and chieftains. One of his long-standing wishes was that he could be a king with all of the absolute power of the kingdom at his disposal. The exploration of this fantasied wish established links to early childhood. I explained to the patient that whereas these kinds of fantasies, which served the purpose of counteracting feelings of helplessness and powerlessness, were relatively safe to have when he was but a small boy, they were now causing him concern. As an adolescent on his way to manhood, he felt he might really be able to implement his wish to exercise power over others, and such fantasies therefore became dangerous.

Another helpful understanding for the patient to have, implied in the preceding discussion, is that his symptoms, discomfiting as they may be, nevertheless serve some purpose for him. They are not adventitious and can therefore be understood and relinquished by him. Strange as it may at first seem to the patient, the troublesome symptom exists because he somewhere feels it to be a lesser evil than those things it helps to keep from his conscious purview.

I have, for example, found it helpful to many patients to explain that people have an automatic and unconscious tendency to expose themselves to dangers essentially identical to those experienced in the past and that, although doing so runs the risk of being hurt once again, this tendency has the important aim of undoing and mastering the trauma of the past. In other words, people tend to actively seek the identical circumstance of the original trauma but with the latent hope that this time they will not suffer the trauma. An important aim of this explanation is to relieve the patient of the feelings of futility, helplessness, and self-depreciation which they experience upon recognizing their repetition of self-destructive behavior.

In Harry's case, this explanation could appropriately be given when he found himself using, inexplicably in a slip of the tongue, the phrase, "whenever I'm hard up for a symptom." He saw the implication that his presumably unwanted and despised symptom was somehow self-engendered, and he was dismayed that he should inflict it on himself. It was proposed that his symptom, even though plaguing, had at the same time the latent aim of mastery over his fear of loss. It was explained that the early fear of loss of parts of his bodily self, his stool and his penis, had apparently been displaced upward to his head and mind in an attempt at solution which had not succeeded. In support of the postulated aim of mastery, it was underscored that his symptom included the aim of regaining his knowledge, a restitution of the feared loss. It was similarly helpful for him to understand, at a later point in the analysis, that the goal of mastery was a factor in the periodic, upsetting recrudescence of his symptoms after they had all but disappeared.

In attempting to convey my understanding of the particular contributions of defense analysis to analytic technique, I have only touched on transference and genetic interpretation. In order to emphasize that defense analysis includes and recognizes the importance of the latter, I shall present one additional excerpt from Harry's analysis.

In the third year of the analysis, Harry's sister went off to college. Despite anticipatory discussion of how this might affect him, Harry found his new situation disturbing. He no longer had his sister as a buffer between himself and his parents, and he was deprived of his essentially masochistic but familiar role of the "little brother." In this role he had to look up to his sister and suffer her domination, but he was compensated for this by her allowing him to be in many ways dependent upon her. In addition, his wishes for freedom, independence, and power were brought closer to realization, and he found this prospect frightening.

For the ensuing two weeks Harry regressed in his behavior and symptoms, and was resistant in the analysis. He then reported the following dream. With the use of scuba equipment, he and a "trio" of middle-aged people were endeavoring to recover some crates containing "bombs or something equally dangerous" from the bottom of the sea. One of the middle-aged persons collapsed and presumably died under water, while the other two, a man and a woman, managed to get up to the surface and out of the ocean, but then collapsed outside of his room at home. He thought these two were dead, but was later told that they only had fainted. He was then suddenly in South America perhaps attending a stage play, but this was vague. The dream shifted again and closed with his mother giving him "hell" for having forgotten his coat and school briefcase, when they were not in fact missing but right there on his seat.

During the day preceding the dream, Harry and his parents had been discussing whether he should go to college in the States or in South America. The latter was his choice because of his intense interest in ancient South American cultures. His parents had suggested that he should talk about this in the analysis. In his usual well-moderated way, he reported his reply as having been, "Why should psychoanalysis, which deals with my sickness, enter into deciding where I go to college?"

The patient's associations to this dream confirmed its rather transparent implications. The analyst was represented by the one in the middle-aged trio who collapsed at the bottom of the sea, and the other two represented his parents. I interpreted that his sister's departure had rekindled his long-standing conflict and anxieties over the freedom but dangers of growing up versus the safety but constrictions of remaining a little boy. It appeared that the "bombs or something equally dangerous" represented that part of himself that he still feared as destructive and uncontrollable if freed. Parenthetically, at an earlier time, we had established that he had so effectively avoided recognition and overt expression of his anger and aggression that he was out of touch with these affects and urges and thus had not learned to modulate them. I had compared his situation in this regard to a radio with a volume control with no positions other than Off or On at full blast.

I further interpreted that he wanted to rid himself of me and his parents as standing in his way, but feared destroying us in the process. I added that the latter possibility was likely given credence in his mind by the deaths of his grandparents. Here, too, it had previously been noted, on the basis of his recollections, that these sudden and inexplicable (to him, at the time) deaths occurred when he had been behaving in a quite free, aggressive, and sometimes obstreperous fashion both in school and at home. We had wondered whether his fantasied explanations of why his grandparents had died included the possibility of a cause and effect relationship between his aggression and their deaths. Linkage to his childhood and the genetic past was gained through the part of the dream in which his mother was giving him hell in an inappropriate way, as if he were still a little boy. In this connection, it was also interpreted that his seeing the analyst and his parents as standing in his way and his fear of destroying us was a kind of replay of what he had apparently felt as a young child: namely, that his mother's actions proved that his aggressive urges and feelings were indeed dangerous and to be feared, disavowed, and denied expression.

SUMMARY AND DISCUSSION

As its title suggests, this paper attempts to demonstrate that the theoretical understanding and technical approach brought to psychoanalysis by ego psychology and defense analysis permits the effective application of the analytic method during adolescence. Because the ego of the adolescent, and particularly the early adolescent, is uniquely threatened by the pubertal surge of instinctual forces, the case of the adolescent is admirably suited for demonstration of defense analysis in its most flexible and extended application. On the other hand, the fact that this presentation is thus weighted in that direction may give the impression that an analyst who values defense analysis is routinely and unduly active in fulfilling its principles to the detriment of other analytic principles such as deprivation in the analytic situation, neutrality, personal anonymity, nonreactiveness, and the sponteneous development of an emotionally charged, analyzable transference. In my experience and to my knowledge, this is not the case. With the aim of being as clear as possible, I shall now in part summarize and reiterate points already made, and in part give some further qualifications.

In my introduction, I mentioned my impression that defense analysis has for many analysts become an integral part of standard technique in the analysis of adults. One might well ask, are not all *Freudian* analyses, by and large, defense analyses; are there alternatives? My own answer would be that they are, and that there are no substantially different alternatives. This is for the reason that the psychoanalytic method has from the beginning recognized a particular kind of defense—unconscious *resistance*—as a central therapeutic issue, and that so much of any analysis deals with resistance in its various forms. Defense analysis includes, however, more than the issue of dealing with resistance. It gives the defensive position of the ego a central prominence in analytic technique, and requires that interpretations be made against the background of a continuing assessment of the total structure of the personality and changes occurring therein, and of the current balance of intrapsychic forces. The aim is to gauge the adequacy of the ego's preparation and tolerance for exposure and interpretation of warded-off unconscious material. The technique emphasizes that we assist the uncovering process in a dynamically meaningful way by focusing simultaneously on the defense and the immediate reasons for it. It places value on expanding the ego's awareness of probable unconscious psychic content and psychic processes as a means of increasing its ability to consciously anticipate that which is feared and threatening from within.

Because every patient is different from every other patient and because the dynamics of each patient are different at different times, the principles of defense analysis are applied upon indication, that is, as and when they are deemed necessary for the progress of the analysis. The indications are both positive and negative, and not simply a matter of last resort. Certain of the techniques or adaptations of technique are relinquished by the analyst as the analytically necessary ego capacities and functions, which formerly had been lacking, develop or return in the patient, and as the ego's tolerance for more direct confrontation with warded-off material increases.

A specific question raised about defense analysis is whether the bypassing of immediately presenting material to focus quite deliberately on some less threatening material can have a negative result. Will the immediately presenting and more threatening material, when thus bypassed, be subjected to tighter repression and become more difficult if not impossible to retrieve? In my experience, this is not the outcome, provided the indication for this temporary bypassing, as based upon the assessment of the contextual situation, has been correct. The intentional use of this technique is quite different, though, from the analyst's unconscious avoidance of, or failure to deal with, presenting material when it is appropriate and even necessary that this be picked up. In other words, it is a matter of awareness and clinical judgment.

The emphasis herein on the need for assessment and judgment—on the analyst's rational processes—in deciding upon the appropriateness of a given technical procedure should not be construed as a devaluation of the analyst's capacity for and use of empathy, intuition, and the analytic ''hunch.'' These capacities in the analyst are vital to the progress and success of any analysis. Defense analysis suggests only that preconscious intuitions and hunches be tested in the analyst's mind against his understanding of the total situation before they are acted upon, something which can under most circumstances be done without interfering with the analytic process.

In presenting and illustrating analytic technique as applied in the case of an early adolescent, I have at the same time been arguing, in effect, that psychoanalysis as a method of treatment should be defined first and fundamentally in terms of its theoretical under-pinnings, its aims, and its methodological requirements, and only secondarily in terms of its technical implementation and the de-velopmental stages and kind of psychopathology to which it can be effectively applied. When psychoanalysis is so defined, the con-strictive effect and the lack of flexibility associated with definition in absolutistic terms are avoided. One can then think -not of conditions to be met a priori and of categorically acceptable or unacceptable techniques, rather, one can think of conditions to be met as soon as possible and of ways for implementing techniques which have been chosen with the aims and requirements of the analytic method constantly in mind and which are compatible with the attainment of analytic goals.

NOTES

[1] In this paper, I am not taking up the question of indications and contraindications for the psychoanalysis of the adolescent (Sklansky, 1972) or the questions of the relevance of the concept and technique of defense analysis to the treatment of the more serious disorders, of analyzability, or of the distinctions between psychoanalysis and psy-choanalytic or dynamic psychotherapy. I am focusing on the concept and technique of defense analysis as it pertains to the psychoanalysis of the adolescent with a neurotic order of psychopathology (Settlage, 1964).

[2]In my usage, the term *defense* includes not only the mechanisms of defense (A. Freud, 1936) but, as here, resistance and other patterns of behavior variously referred to as a defensive position, posture, or stance.

[3]As Gill (1963, Chapters 5 and 6) noted in his discussion of the theoretical bases for the technique of defense analysis, the clearest and most comprehensive presentation of the early evolution of this technique is that of Fenichel (1941). Since then, contributions focused pointedly on the relationship between defense organization and psychoanalytic technique have been made by Hartmann (1951), Eissler (1953), Loewenstein (1954), Hoffer (1954), Weiss (1971), and in the panels reported by Zetzel (1954) and Pumpian-Mindlin (1967). In addition, pertinent contributions, although not focused directly on the subject, have been made by Bornstein (1949), Loewenstein (1956), and Harley (1962).

[4]This point is nicely illustrated in Harley's (1970) work with early adolescents, set forth in a paper which also provides understanding of important nuances in the psychology of early adolescent development.

[5]Gill (1953) gave the following description: "The progressive analysis of defense often sets out from the conscious, ego-syntonic content, which becomes exposed as a defense against preconscious defensive contents which attain consciousness with some difficulty, and which, in turn, are exposed as defenses against more primitive unconscious defenses whose organization shows some primary-process characteristics" (p. 123).

[6]As Mahler (1968) has elucidated, psychogenetically significant libidinal loss can be experienced by the child even though the mother continues to be physically present in the environment. One of the most obvious situations in which this occurs is that of postpartum depression. The depressed mother may be quite capable of ministering to the physical and physiologic needs of the child while at the same time being withdrawn from him emotionally.

[7]The concept that separation-individuation is revisited and reworked in the context of each successive state of development was discussed by the author at the December 1971 meetings of the American Psychoanalytic Association as a member of the panel on The Experience of Separation-Individuation in Infancy and Its Reverberations throughout the Course of Life: 1. Infancy and Childhood (Winestine, 1973).

[8]Although illustrated in work with borderline and psychotic children, the technique of allowing the patient to maintain psychological distance

from too threatening material was, to my knowledge, first reported by Ekstein and Wallerstein (1956) in their discussion of metaphoric interpretation. The term is used by both Harley (1962) and Maenchen (1970) in their discussion of the analysis of neurotic children and adolescents.

[9]The latter material raises the important question of the genesis and role of the ego ideal during childhood development and particularly during adolescence. For a discussion of this question, see Settlage (1972), Cultural values and the superego in late adolescence, *Psychoanalytic Study of the Child* 27:74-92. New Haven, Yale University Press.

[10]Such explanations are given in a natural and contextual way, using technical terms when their meaning would be clear to the patient and using equivalent words or language when this would not be the case.

BIBLIOGRAPHY

Blos, P. 1967. The second individuation process of adolescence. *Psychoanalytic Study of the Child* 22:162-86.

Bornstein, B. 1949. The analysis of a phobic child. *Psychoanalytic Study of the Child* 3-4:181-226.

Brenner, C. 1957. The value and development of the concept of repression in Freud's writings. *Psychoanalytic Study of the Child* 12:19-46.

Casuso, G. 1965. The relationship between child analysis and the theory and practice of adult analysis. Panel Report in *Journal of the American Psychoanalytic Association* 13:159-71.

Eissler, K. R. 1953. The effect of the structure of the ego on psychoanalytic technique. *Journal of the American Psychoanalytic Association* 1:104-43.

————. 1958. Notes on problems of technique in the psychoanalytic treatment of adolescents. *Psychoanalytic Study of the Child* 13:223-54.

Ekstein, R., and Wallerstein, J. 1956. Observations on the psychotherapy of borderline and psychotic children. *Psychoanalytic Study of the Child* 11:303-11.

Fenichel, O. 1941. *Problems of psychoanalytic technique*. Albany, N.Y.: Psychoanalytic Quarterly.

―――. 1945. *The psychoanalytic theory of neurosis*. New York: W. W. Norton.

Freud, A. 1936. *The ego and the mechanisms of defence*. New York: International Universities Press, 1946.

―――. 1958. Adolescence. *Psychoanalytic Study of the Child* 13:255-78.

Freud, S. 1923. The ego and the id. *Standard edition* 19:3-66. London: Hogarth Press, 1961.

Group for the Advancement of Psychiatry, Committee on Adolescence (GAP6). 1968. *Normal adolescence: Its dynamics and impact*, Report No. 68. New York: Charles Scribner's Sons.

Geleerd, E. R. 1957. Some aspects of psychoanalytic technique in adolescence. *Psychoanalytic Study of the Child* 12:263-83.

Gill, M.M. 1963. *Topography and systems in psychoanalytic theory*. Psychological Issues, Monograph 10. New York: International Universities Press.

Harley, M. 1962. The role of the dream in the analysis of a latency child. *Journal of the American Psychoanalytic Association* 10:271-88.

―――. 1970. On some problems of technique in the analysis of early adolescents. *Psychoanalytic Study of the Child* 25:99-121.

Hartmann, H. 1939. *Ego psychology and the problem of adaptation*. New York: International Universities Press.

―――. 1951. Technical implications of ego psychology. *Psychoanalytic Quarterly* 20:31-43.

Hoffer, W. 1954. Defensive process and defensive organization: Their place in psycho-analytic technique. *International Journal of Psycho-Analysis* 23:194-98.

Loewenstein, R.M. 1954. Some remarks on defenses, autonomous ego, and psycho-analytic technique. *International Journal of Psycho-Analysis* 35:188-93.

―――. 1956. Some remarks on the role of speech in psycho-analytic technique. *International Journal of Psycho-Analysis* 37:460-68.

―――. 1967. Defensive organization and autonomous ego functions. *Journal of the American Psychoanalytic Association* 15:795-809.

Maenchen, A. 1970. On the technique of child analysis in relation to stages of development. *Psychoanalytic Study of the Child* 25:175-208.

Mahler, M.S. 1965. On the significance of the normal separation-individuation phase: With reference to research in symbiotic child psychosis. In *Drives, affects, behavior*, ed. M. Schur, vol. 2, pp. 161-69. New York: International Universities Press.

————. 1968. *On human symbiosis and the vicissitudes of individuation*, vol. 1, *Infantile psychosis*. New York: International Universities Press.

Pumpian-Mindlin, E. 1967. Defensive organization of the ego and psychoanalytic technique. Panel report in *Journal of the American Psychoanalytic Association* 15:150-65.

Reich, W. 1933. *Character-analysis*, 3rd ed. New York: Orgone Institute Press, 1949.

Settlage, C.F. 1964. Psychoanalytic theory in relation to the nosology of childhood psychic disorders. *Journal of the American Psychoanalytic Association* 12:776-89.

————. 1971. On the libidinal aspect of early psychic development and the genesis of the infantile neurosis. In *Separation-Individuation: Essays in honor of Margaret S. Mahler*, ed. J.B. McDevitt and C.F. Settlage, pp. 131-54. New York: International Universities Press.

Sklansky, M.A. 1972. Indications and contraindications for the psychoanalysis of the adolescent. Panel report in *Journal of the American Psychoanalytic Association* 20:134-44.

Weiss, J. 1971. The emergence of new themes: A contribution to the psycho-analytic theory of therapy. *International Journal of Psycho-Analysis* 52:459-67.

Winestine, M. C. 1973. The experience of operation-individuation in infancy and its reverberations throught the course of life: I. Infancy and childhood. Panel Report in *Journal of American Psychoanalytic Association* 21:135-154.

Zetzel, E.R. 1954. Defense mechanisms and psychoanalytic technique. Panel Report in *Journal of the American Psychoanalytic Association* 2:318-26.

Treatment of a Bisexual Conflict in Prepuberty and Adolescence

Elizabeth Daunton   *Cleveland*

Bruce, the elder of identical twins, began analysis shortly before his eleventh birthday. His parents were distressed by his feminine interests and a long-standing symptom of dressing up in his mother's or sisters' underwear or jewelry. Bruce had begun to do this when he was 4 years old. The parents had first discussed the problem with the family doctor when Bruce was 6 but no further action was taken at this time. Three years later, the parents requested a psychiatric evaluation for Bruce; their concern about the learning difficulties of his twin, Bill, led to an evaluation of both boys, and analysis was recommended and accepted for each twin.

The first two years of Bruce's analysis took place before he had reached puberty. This period of work was most revealing about his defenses, his pre-oedipal relationship with his mother, and his thoughts and feelings about his twinship and his relations with Bill. I shall present some material from this phase of the treatment, hoping thereby to convey something of its flavor ·as well as the light that was shed thus far on Bruce's symptom and on his internal conflicts.

As Bruce entered adolescence, his castration anxiety came into

From the Department of Psychiatry, University Hospitals, Case Western Reserve University, Cleveland, Ohio.

I wish to thank Dr. Anny Katan, Professor Emeritus of Child Analysis, Case Western Reserve University for her helpful discussion of this patient in her Child Analysis Seminar.

sharper focus and was now painfully experienced. I could then understand more clearly how Bruce had tried to bind the castration anxiety through his transvestite symptom. Some analytic work from the adolescent phase of the analysis will be presented in greater detail.

PRESENTING PROBLEM AND HISTORY

Bruce's parents had been frightened and embarrassed by his symptom. They recalled that at first he had paraded before the family in female clothes as though hoping to be admired. Instead, his parents had scolded and occasionally had spanked Bruce while his brothers and sisters had teased him. Bruce was hurt and bewildered by this treatment and had become sullen and tearful. For approximately a year before his referral, the parents had tried to restrain their anger with Bruce; they had discouraged his teasing by the other children and had tried to show special interest in his achievements. He then had become more ashamed of his problem and had gained greater control of it, although periodically he still took an item of clothing or jewelry into his own room. He tried to disguise his liking for his sisters' dolls while maintaining a strong interest in female fashions.

A boy of average ability, Bruce had some difficulties in learning. He misread words, was an indifferent speller, and could not express himself easily in writing. In general, his teachers liked him and thought he got on well with his classmates. Bruce avoided sports in which his twin excelled; swimming was the one area where he had pleasure and success. Outside school, his company was not sought by other boys; at best they tolerated him as the companion of his popular twin.

Bruce's mother was a warm, attractive woman with a good sense of humor. She had high expectations of herself as a mother and strong guilt when she felt she did not fulfill them. As I came to know her better, I found her an excellent observer of her children and unusually sensitive to their feelings. The reality events in the mother's life were often overwhelming; she tended to deal with unconscious anxiety by becoming very angry and then suffering from self-reproach. The twins' relatively poor school achievement resulted in her marked irritation with them because she felt she had not given them as much as she had given her other children, who were good students. I was impressed by the mother, in an early interview, when she reflected that there could be a link between Bruce having begun to wear her clothes at age 4 and her preoccupation, in the previous months, with his twin, who had been seriously ill for a long period.

The father was a hard-working man, interested in each of his children. He had rather low self-esteem and talked in a joking, deprecating way about himself. He was sorry for Bruce, as well as embarrassed by him, and felt bad that he was, himself, more in tune with Bill and his eldest son, who shared his own interest in sports. He identified with Bill, who had fears similar to his own as a child, and who handled them in a similar way.

Bruce's mother had been completely unprepared for the birth of twins. She recalled having been pleased by other people's interest but having found their care most burdensome. She reproached herself for not having as much time to love the twins as her other babies, but had found comfort in the belief that the twins provided company for each other and therefore needed less of her time. Although she could observe certain differences in temperament and achievement between them in the first year, the mother could not reliably tell the twins apart until their fifth year, when their differences in personality became more pronounced. It was difficult for the mother, therefore, to recall separate milestones in the twins' development. Only their different medical experiences were firmly etched in her memory. The mother was unhappy that she had not been able to breast feed the twins. They had been weaned gradually from bottle to cup at 18 months; weaning had not been easy but the mother had felt that it was important not to hurry the twins. Both babies had presented some health problems in their first year. Bill had an operative procedure when he was a month old. Both boys had inguinal hernias which were treated with trusses; Bruce wore his until he was 9 months old. The twins sat up at about 6 months, began walking at 13 months. Bill was the more active and lively, Bruce the more placid of the two.

Perhaps because they could receive less time and stimulation from the mother, the twins began to talk much later than their brothers and sisters. They attempted single words at 18 months and began to speak in sentences at 3. Both had a slight lisp and their speech was indistinct when they began school at 5. They had speech therapy at 6 and responded quickly to individual help.

The twins' toilet training proved most taxing to the mother's patience. She described it as difficult and inconsistent. She had begun training the twins at one year but "had given up" after several months of unsuccessful coaxing. Training had begun again before the twins' second birthday. At this point, the mother had strapped the boys on the toilet, as they were unwilling to sit there for more than brief moments. The mother recalled that at times she had been very permissive about soiling and wetting; at other times, she would get angry, raise her voice, and sometimes spank. Both twins were trained for bowel movements by about 2-1/2 but were not reliably dry by day or night until after their fourth birthday. At about this time, there had been a change in the family sleeping arrangements. Until they were 4, the twins had slept in the parents' room. They then moved to a room of their own where they shared a double bed. There was a casual attitude to privacy in the home.

Bruce had his first separation from his mother at 2, when his sister Susan was born. The mother could not remember how the twins had reacted to her absence or to the birth of their sister. During their fourth year, the twins had their first and only long separation from each other, when Bill became seriously ill with an acute infection. As he maintained a high fever, he was admitted to the hospital for tests and observation; he remained in the hospital for a month and required another month's careful nursing by his mother at home. I do not know how much explanation Bruce was given at the time about Bill's illness. Looking back, the mother recognized that Bruce must have felt deeply the separation from Bill, the parents' worry and preoccupation, and the loss of his mother's company.

Bruce had many difficult experiences in the following years. When he was 4, he fell from a fence, cutting his head; the cut was closed by stitches in the emergency room of the hospital. His mother became pregnant again during the same year. The twins asked the mother about her pregnancy; she was glad to discuss it with them and prepare them for the birth of the baby. Their sister, Kathy, was born when the twins were 5. In the same year, both twins had tonsillectomies; their mother remained with them and they did not stay overnight at the hospital.

When Bruce was 8, his mother had a miscarriage which she was able to discuss with the children. The following year, she developed a serious physical illness and had to leave home for the hospital on the day of the twins' birthday party. After her return home, she was confined to bed for three months. A close relative helped to care for the family at this time.

BRUCE'S TREATMENT IN PREPUBERTY

My early impressions of Bruce were of a nice-looking, slightly plump boy whose short stature made him look about a year younger than his age. Although very neatly dressed, he did not make an effeminate impression; he did have an unusual walk, moving very quietly with short, quick steps. He always greeted me and spoke with other people in the waiting room in a quiet, polite manner. At times when he felt comfortable in the office, he had a pleasant smile and expression. At other times, he showed that he was lost in fantasy by a faraway look in his eyes and a blank expression.

Having treatment with a different analyst from his brother's, and coming to a separate building, placed Bruce in an unusual situation. I first became aware of how strange Bruce felt and how much he missed his twin's support when he told me of an experience he shared with Bill, on their morning paper route. This gave me a chance to explore with Bruce how he felt about coming separately for treatment. I learned that the twins were experiencing another separation concurrently. They had shared a bed since they were 4 and now were to have single ones. While consciously Bruce looked forward to the change, unconsciously he experienced a feeling of loss. The new beds were to come at the time of the twins' birthday, when I had said I would give Bruce a gift. He asked me for a teddy bear, explaining that Bill and he had owned toy dogs ever since they had been small; now the dogs were hard to cuddle because their insides were coming out. Bruce was most disappointed that I gave him another gift instead of the teddy bear. In discussing his disappointment, I suggested that he might have wanted the bear to help him get over the separation from Bill both in treatment and at bedtime. Bruce replied that when they were 5 they used to cuddle together to keep warm, showing that his separation feelings could so far only be recognized in terms of the past.

Helping Bruce to understand treatment was a difficult task because he feared that I would punish or ridicule him if he shared his problems with me. His first reference to his problem was expressed by a projection: he said that he had wondered if I would wear "funny" clothes since I came from another country. A chance to discuss his fear of being misunderstood, and his sense of bewilderment, came when Bruce volunteered that he used to take girls' parts in plays. He explained, with a sheepish smile, that he had taken these parts because his Cub Scout leader had thought he was good at them; his mother had not wanted him to take these parts, nor had he, himself, wanted to. When I remarked that Bruce did not want to upset his mother, he replied, "When I was about 6,

I used to play with dolls, I used to be a tomgirl, I mean a tomboy.''
He went on to complain that the boys at school still called him a
sissy, just because he liked a girl in his class. Bruce's slip showed
me his wish to admit his problem, which he could not do openly,
however, because of his fear of my reaction. I replied that it was as
though he had two pictures of himself, one more like a tomboy and
the other a tomgirl. I went on to say that he might expect me to be
angry with him, as his family had been, if he showed interest in
girls' things. Perhaps he was not sure whether it was better to be a
''tomboy or tomgirl'' because of many worries he had had in his
life; I would like the chance to help him understand these worries
better.

It took a long time for Bruce to derive any reassurance from such
comments. For many months, when I referred to some aspect of
his bisexual conflict, he would react sullenly or with a sudden
outburst of anger. I had often to remark that he became angry to
protect himself from the anger he expected from me. Bruce had
also internal prohibitions about certain activities which he showed
in an interesting way in his early sessions. He appeared fascinated
by the toys in my office but did not investigate or play with them.
In reply to my inquiry, he said he did not think I would allow play
and added that he could not allow it, himself. On further reflection,
he thought that his mother would not like it. Bruce agreed when I
asked whether he felt that this would be like playing with his
sisters' toys. After I had explained the reason for having toys in the
office, and had suggested that he might want to discuss this with
his mother, Bruce played with the toys from time to time. I then
noticed that sometimes Bruce would abruptly get up from his chair
after a period of talking and move over to the toy table. Bruce
explained, ''I must spend part of my time talking here, though I'd
like to play; after I've controlled myself for a while, then I feel I'm
allowed to play.'' In this way, Bruce revealed his unconscious
masturbation conflict which was not discussed at this early stage of

treatment. Later, this conflict could be linked with his learning difficulty.

When treatment began, Bruce's mother was in the ninth month of a pregnancy. Further, it was only six weeks before Christmas when I planned to take a week's vacation.[1] Bruce showed feelings of concern for his mother in our discussions, but her pregnancy and his brother's birth also stirred up feelings with which he had to deal defensively. These were feelings of loneliness, fear of loss of love, envy and the anger associated with these painful affects.

During the last phase of his mother's pregnancy, confinement, and return home, I gradually became acquainted with Bruce's defenses, which were prominent, too, when we discussed the approaching vacation. Bruce's memory was greatly disturbed by repression; he could not remember events in sequence or whether something had occurred recently or last year. I should like also to stress Bruce's use of identification and denial because these defenses played so prominent a role in his disturbance. Much work was needed to help Bruce recognize his denial of his problem with his schoolwork. For many months, he could see his difficulties but fleetingly and only when he received his report card. Even then, he could not "look at" his problems to see what the difficulties were; he merely castigated himself and resolved to do better.

When the baby was overdue, Bruce identified with his mother by taking a long time to produce a thought and by heavy silences in his hour; before then, he had been rather talkative. In his appointment after the birth, he spoke of his ambition to lose weight as well as his fear of being given the same anesthesia by the dentist as had been administered to his mother. Bruce's use of denial could be approached through his understanding of his mother's defensive joking about her size when the baby was overdue. When I said, "I think mother jokes to help her stand a worry," Bruce compared these times with "the old days when mothers had their babies at home and sometimes died because they didn't get looked after well.'' ''The old days'' for Bruce were not long ago. He spoke next of his mother having lost her last baby and thought this was because she had been so ill the year before. When I said that this must have been a very worrisome time for him, Bruce thought of Little Orphan Annie and explained that, ''orphanages are for children whose mothers have died and whose fathers can't take care of them.''

Bruce had isolated the anxious feelings connected with his mother's last absence: he did not remember any worries, he recalled only the dates. In another hour, he spoke again about his mother's health and asked me for a realistic explanation of her illness. When I had given it, he revealed his fantasy that by being a twin he had harmed his mother. He reflected that his mother might now be carrying twins, ''because it's taking so long.'' He thought more time was needed for a twin pregnancy, ''because the mother has to become more pregnant and fatter.'' I asked if he knew how his mother's pregnancy had been in relation to his and Bill's birth. Bruce replied that she had become very big and could hardly walk because he and Bill were so heavy. Bruce agreed when I said that he felt he had harmed his mother by being born a twin, and that feeling responsible would make it hard for him to believe that she was well enough to have the baby she was expecting now.

Although Bruce had been told by his mother that his treatment would last for more than a year, he pressed me both before and after my vacation to tell him exactly when it would end, anticipating that it would be in a few weeks' time. He was evidently afraid of being taken by surprise, although his conscious thought was that he only came to treatment to please his mother. However, Bruce began to have some fantasies about other patients and became very much concerned about gifts which he might exchange at Christmas. After quoting his mother's joking remark that she would have to have another baby just when she had ''got rid'' of the other kids in school, Bruce imagined that before his hour I had been looking at a list of names so that I could choose his successor. When we discussed this, he could easily recognize his idea that I planned to get rid of him, but he could not recognize the feelings which accompanied this thought.

As Christmas approached, Bruce showed his interest in female clothes by talking of the presents he would like to give me. He had thought of a sweater, hose, or a slip, and I learned that he paid close attention to what I wore. Boys' clothes were mentioned as possible gifts for him. The clothes Bruce wished to give me were ones his mother liked to receive; Bruce recalled, too, that the previous year his father had given his mother a nice fur. He added that many women are too free with their husband's money and that if he were a husband he would not allow this.

Bruce's preoccupation with clothes, whether his own or other people's, struck me as most unusual for a boy in prepuberty and guided me in my thinking about him. It might seem that in wishing to give me clothes, Bruce was identifying with his father. However, his unusual interest in these clothes, combined with his thought that women were not always deserving, suggested rather that he was warding off a wish to be treated like his mother by the use of a passive into active defense. This meant that instead of entertaining the wish to be given female clothes, he thought of giving them to me. At this stage in the treatment, Bruce was convinced that he no longer had his transvestite symptom; to have interpreted his defense would therefore have aroused an intolerable anxiety. Because I thought his longing for love was nearer to consciousness than his defense, I replied to his thoughts about his mother's gifts by saying that these were a sign of love and that Bruce might well wish to have such a valuable sign of love from his father. Bruce agreed ruefully, and with some resentment, that he felt both his mother and sisters got more love from his father than did he.

Bruce indicated the connection between the exchange of gifts and the approaching separation in an acting out in the transference. This acting out occurred before the last appointment preceding the vacation. The acting out also threw light on Bruce's relationship with his twin. Bruce's defenses became stronger as we approached the holidays. He forgot when they were to begin and apologized that he could not come on Christmas Eve when there was no scheduled appointment. In the next to last hour before the holiday, Bruce brought some candy for me. It became clear that he was afraid that I would not give him a present after all, although I had said I would do so on the following day. His associations were that it was the girls and small children who were lucky at Christmas. "Only" children, like his cousin, also did better. In talking of this cousin, Bruce made a slip, calling him a "*lonely*" child. I suggested that I was like the lucky girl who had her gift and he was like the unlucky, lonely boy.

Between this appointment and the last one before the holidays, Bruce visited a drug store with another boy and became interested in a pair of earrings. It appeared that, at Bruce's suggestion, the other boy had taken them and had presented them to his mother. This mother reported the incident to Bruce's parents who encouraged Bruce to return the earrings to the store. Bruce did not mention this incident in his last appointment before the holidays. He expressed great pleasure at my gift, and told me next that Bill had received a gift from his analyst two days previously. I was impressed to learn that Bruce had not consciously perceived this gift at first, even though Bill had displayed it in their bedroom.

I learned about the earring incident from Bruce's mother after the vacation, but Bruce, himself, made no reference to it. When I referred to it, Bruce acted in an angry, defensive way. He did not mean to mention it, he said, because, "It's all over and done with." I suggested that once again Bruce might worry that to share a trouble would lead to my getting angry; better to prevent that by keeping quiet. I thought that, instead of getting angry, it was better to try to understand the hidden feelings which got him into trouble. Bruce then gave his account of what had happened at the store. He had picked up the earrings, intending to give them to his mother but he could not get the attention of the lady to wait on him "because she was busy with someone else"; so then he had suggested that his friend take them without paying. When I commented that this had happened the day before the vacation, when Bruce had expressed the feeling that I was getting rid of him for someone else, Bruce replied that he did not care at all about the vacation. I interpreted that he must have felt that I was like the lady in the store, too busy to care about his needs. I also linked his "left out feelings" attendant on his mother's need to give much time to the baby with his "left out feelings" when Bill was given his gift first by his analyst. Bruce then recalled that our vacation had begun on a Friday which reminded him of other Friday separations. His mother had gone to the hospital to have Kathy on a Friday and had returned home a week later. When I linked his "missing feelings" at that time with his recent vacation feelings, Bruce looked very sad.

From later remarks about my earrings which Bruce associated with those in the store, I understood that he had really wanted the earrings himself as a way of managing his feelings of loss. This further suggested the meaning of Bruce's transvestite symptom at one level. In wearing something connected with his mother, he dealt with anxiety about losing her care and attention by identification (A. Freud, 1965).

A theoretical question at this time was whether Bruce was displacing conflicts in his current life about the new baby rather than experiencing a transference conflict, with its roots in the past. I concluded that he had "acted out in the transference" because his current unconscious feelings about his mother were largely dealt with by identification, while those about me had been repressed. As they became conscious to Bruce, through analysis of the acting out, he associated them with previous, painful experiences of loss. Of course, these old conflicts had been strongly reactivated by the recent events in Bruce's life: his mother's hospitalization and his brother's birth. Twice later during the treatment, Bruce took small items, once from a store and once from my office. Both times, Bruce was warding off feelings of disappointment, anger, and guilt. One incident was directly linked with an illness of his baby brother, and the other was a reaction in the transference. As Bruce became more conscious of painful guilt feelings, he discussed the incidents spontaneously in the analysis and made restitution of his own accord.

Further material showed that both the transference feeling of rejection and the feeling that Bill was preferred by his analyst were rooted in the early mother-twin relationship. They had been reinforced when his sisters had been born and even more in his fourth year, when Bill's illness had led to a disturbance of his relationship both with his mother and with his twin. Currently, Bruce was beginning to take an active part in the care of his baby brother, Peter. He enjoyed feeding and changing Peter, but he became anxious when the baby cried in the early morning and would go to the parents' room to try to soothe him. Peter had an inguinal hernia which was repaired when he was four months old.

Bruce's identification with his mother in her anxiety was most revealing and could be traced to her early mothering of Bill. Bruce showed his concern by worrying about a boy he had seen near my office and who, he supposed, was my patient. This boy had severe tics and Bruce described him as a very nervous boy. I asked if he knew any other nervous boys, which led Bruce to tell how much Peter cried because of his hernia. He then spoke of conversations he had heard about Bill's illness as a small baby. I remarked that Bruce might feel that I was more concerned about a patient who was sicker and more nervous than himself. Bruce then related what he both had heard and imagined about the way in which he and Bill had been fed as small babies. He thought Bill had been breast fed longer "because he was weaker and I had to make do with cows' milk, which is short on vitamins." This fantasy, a number of cover memories, and his intense feelings of rejection in the transference convinced me that Bruce's feelings of deprivation had begun in the triangular relationship of the first year.[2] Further material showed that the identification with the mother's anxiety was reinforced by Bill's illness in the fourth year. When Bill currently went for physical check-ups, which were not necessary for Bruce, Bruce accompanied Bill; he was unaware of his concern about Bill's health, claiming, "I just go along for the ride."

A striking feature of Bruce's analysis was his avoidance of speaking about his body and its functions. His reticence exceeded by far the usual shyness and modesty and seemed to be caused by a strong inhibition in thinking about his body. His interest in his own and other people's bodies had been diverted to an unusually strong interest and pleasure in clothes. He had given one clue, near the beginning of treatment, that this avoidance was linked with castration fears. He described the hospital building where he had had his tonsillectomy as "one for the upper part of you; eyes, nose, throat." When I mentioned, from time to time, that he seemed shy about mentioning his body, Bruce became stubbornly defensive.

In the second year of treatment, it became possible to understand how anal conflicts had contributed both to Bruce's inhibition and to his learning difficulties. Before a vacation, Bruce spoke of having read about a woman who wanted her baby adopted because she was tired of washing diapers. Another day he said, with embarrassment, that he had thought I was in the bathroom when he had come for his appointment. He then remembered a time when he and Bill had stayed on a farm when they had been small, recalling vividly the dirtiness of the animals, especially the pigs, "who walked in dirt and ate garbage." I now discussed with Bruce what I knew about the difficulties of his toilet training, suggesting that he might have thought as a small boy that he and Bill had been sent away from home for being dirty. I went on to suggest that one reason for his shyness in talking about body matters with me could be his worry that I would say this talk was bad or dirty, or perhaps even send him away.[3]

Several authors[4] have stressed how difficult it is for an identical twin to develop a clear self-image and see himself as a separate person, able to function in his own right. The physical closeness with his twin and the availability of the twin as an object for identification contribute to his difficulty. In a number of ways, Bruce showed that, for him, the boundaries between himself and Bill were sometimes indistinct. One day he spoke of being grown-up with the qualification "if I live that long." When I asked what could prevent it, he replied that he might get killed by a car. He then recalled that once Bill had been crossing the street and had not noticed a truck until he was a few yards away. Bruce was following and had been scared lest Bill run into the truck. When I remarked that his fear for Bill was now felt as fear for himself, Bruce remembered his mother having had a car accident; in this way he indicated that the boundaries between himself, twin, and mother were not always clear and that both mother and twin were ready objects of identification. This example shows, too, how difficulties to individuation and ready use of identification served to heighten Bruce's castration anxiety. As treatment progressed, Bruce revealed an increasing wish to delineate himself clearly as a person in his own right. This aim was nicely expressed in his proud description of his bicycle as "just one of a kind."

It was also interesting to trace the effects of the twin relationship on Bruce's superego formation. He was a boy whose ego ideal contained high standards of courtesy and social decorum. At times, Bruce's inner controls seemed more effective than Bill's, at others he tried to master his own unconscious impulses by censorship of Bill, criticizing him severely for smoking or swearing. There were also times when Bruce could not always trust his own controls, and when he then looked to Bill for reinforcement. One day before a vacation from treatment, he expressed the fear that he might be tempted to steal when he went downtown. He decided to ask Bill to accompany him, explaining, "He knows how to behave." While Bruce had an internalized superego, the twin relationship, which was so readily available for projections and identifications, made it harder for him to rely with confidence on his own superego as his own independent guide.

Internal conflicts, rooted in masculine and feminine strivings, now came to the fore in the analytic work. It was apparent that Bruce could not allow himself masculine goals because these led to feelings of hopelessness in respect to competing with Bill, and aroused intense castration anxiety. Bruce associated his reluctance to play football to injuries he had received as a small boy. He vividly recalled having gone to the emergency room to have his scalp stitched after falling from a fence. He remembered being intensely afraid and thought that "he had blanked out" while the stitches were being put in. He thought that his mother had been with him and that the worst part had been when she had left to call his father. Bruce could accept my suggestion that when he got cuts or bruises at football, the fear he experienced was so great because it belonged to his early, frightening experience.

In the spring, Bruce made some attempt to take part in baseball; he could neither enjoy it nor achieve success at it. Later, he felt hopeless about playing basketball because Bill did much better and won praise and prestige for his skill. While Bruce consciously envied Bill's success, unconsciously he feared that were he to compete with Bill, this would destroy his brother. This fear arose from his intense aggression toward Bill, which he warded off by isolation and displacement.

At this time, Bruce conveyed some aggressive fantasies through doll play in the office. Members of a doll family were run over by cars and beaten up. Bruce was indignant when I eventually suggested that some feelings about members of his own family might be shown in these games. His indignation sprang from his fear of loss of control and from his magical thinking. When we discussed how hard it was to recognize some of our own feelings, Bruce volunteered, "I'm often mad at my brothers, but I don't want to hurt them." We discussed Bruce's fear that anger must lead to loss of control and this then paved the way for my later interpretation that Bruce feared getting hurt in sports because of his aggressive wishes about Bill or, at other times, his father. Bruce also had the fantasy that Bill's "skinniness" was due to his "getting mad." Conversely, he thought that by "keeping my anger in," he could remain superior in weight and strength to Bill.

The other side of Bruce's inhibition in sports was seen in his envy of Bill's shared interest with his father in this area. Competing in sports meant not only a dangerous competition with Bill, and ultimately with his father, but also competition with Bill for his father's approval. When Bruce enrolled in a class in order to have a separate summer activity from Bill's, the same conflict emerged. At first, all went well, but soon Bruce complained that the teacher was losing interest in him and paying more attention to other students. Bruce now experienced with his father and teachers the same feelings of narcissistic injury and loss that had formed part of his early relationship with the mother. At this stage in his treatment, he was often late for his appointment because it was painful to see and compare himself with another patient. He also expressed resentment that Bill's analyst admired his skill in sports and consequently, he thought, had a poor opinion of Bruce. Bruce's fear of competition with Bill was also noticeable in his school-work. He was proud of being more conscientious and getting somewhat better grades but did not want "to get too far ahead."

Arlo (1960) has shown that the order of birth is most meaningful to twins and contributes richly to their fantasies. While Bruce's schoolwork was under discussion, he stressed that he was the first born and spoke with pride of having been born just two minutes and eighteen seconds before Bill. I replied by suggesting that he seemed to want to keep just this little way ahead of Bill in his schoolwork. We could gradually recognize, then, that Bruce's difficulty in working freely and uninfluenced by Bill's performance sprang from his guilt over his rivalry with Bill.

While, in the first year of treatment, Bruce quickly withdrew from competitive situations in which he felt less favored and adequate than his twin, he handled his negative oedipal wishes in a different way by identifications which were well tolerated by his ego. On two occasions, he wore a ring to his session. The first time followed his parents' wedding anniversary. I learned that the ring had been lent to Bruce by his elder brother to whom the father had given it. Bruce reflected about the gifts which were appropriate for various anniversaries. I remarked that a wedding ring is the first gift which a husband gives his wife, and suggested that his interest in the ring showed his great longing to be loved by his father as was his mother.

Bruce also wore a ring on his mother's birthday and again thought of the gifts of clothes and money that his mother had received from his father. Further material indicated his envy of his mother for being able to have babies. This could be seen in his behavior with Peter; he would willingly have taken over the complete care of his little brother. Bruce could not master all these feelings by identification. When rivalrous feelings with his mother became too strong, they were displaced to his sisters and their dolls. He spoke angrily of his elder sister, who would not let anyone play with her dolls, "because she is saving them for her own children."

In the transference, Bruce questioned whether I bought my own clothes or whether they were given me by a man. When I cancelled two appointments to attend meetings Bruce wondered whether I would buy new clothes, which would be a way of showing off and attracting attention. After my return, Bruce imagined that I had "stayed at a hotel and gone out with the girls." He denied any further interest but showed that my absence had stimulated both his envy and passive excitement by relating the plots of two movies, *I Was a Teenage Werewolf* and *King Kong*. He described how King Kong had chased a girl to the window ledge of her hotel room where she had been rescued from him by her fiance. I commented that the movie plots were most exciting compared with the dull time he thought I had had; could he have preferred me to have had a dull time because he was afraid of the opposite? Perhaps thinking that I had spent time with a man would make him feel too excited and envious. Bruce found it hard to accept this, but I now learned that before the cancelled appointments he had taken a small doll from the office and had used some of his mother's jewelry to dress up one of his sisters' dolls. I could now discuss with Bruce that it was at times when he felt envious of his mother or me, and wished that he were "in our shoes," that he felt he must acquire a doll baby for himself.

Bruce and his brother often engaged in bedtime roughhousing. While Bruce described the aim of the bouts as "to get each other down" he denied both the angry and excited aspects of the play. It became clear, however, that Bruce had a variety of defenses with which to keep his passive excitement unconscious. Some of these were detrimental to his relationships in that friendly feelings, which might lead to excitement, were defended against by resentful, disgruntled feelings. When Bruce went out with boys in the neighborhood, he looked forward to the occasions but something always went wrong. If they made a trip downtown, it would be spoiled because the other boys had plans different from his own. His warded-off excitement was more apparent when Bruce described games of chasing with other boys in which he was usually being pursued. In this period, hours in which Bruce was quite friendly were often followed by hours in which he would be sullen and irritated by treatment, and when he would come late for appointments. It occurred to me that Bruce became negative to me for the same reason that he became negative to his friends; warm friendly feelings were too much involved with excitement to be tolerated. This hypothesis was confirmed when I learned more about Bruce's practice of switching on the light as he entered the office every day, even when there was bright sunshine. I learned that he did not like dark rooms and that his evaluation interview with a male psychiatrist had taken place in a room which "was much too dark.'' Bruce remembered having been very frightened of this doctor who, he thought, might kidnap him. When I asked how the doctor had behaved, Bruce replied, ''he was friendly, smiled at me and put his feet on the table.''

During this time, when Bruce was frequently dissatisfied with me and his treatment, we arranged to miss an hour so that he could take a school test. The following day, he expressed anger about the cancelled appointment; the test had not been given but by then it had been too late to come. I could now discuss with Bruce how he became dissatisfied with me and the boys he knew when he really wanted to be friendly with us. I thought that he had to turn his feelings right around because he was so afraid that being friendly would mean getting excited together. This interpretation helped Bruce to be more open about mutually exciting play between himself and Bill. It also paved the way to understanding the link between Bruce's guilt and some of his learning difficulties. He observed closely the way other children left materials in the office, and he criticized me for allowing another patient to leave crayon marks on my desk. At this time, Bruce was himself provoking his teacher to scold him for incompleted work and was fearful that his father would punish him for a poor report card. I suggested that Bruce was asking for the punishment from his father and teacher that he thought I should give to children in the office for messy, out-of-control behavior. This seeking of punishment could be linked both with the exciting play with his brother and with his own masturbation. Learning became more neutralized for Bruce and his interest in it increased after he could recognize that displacement of these conflicts onto school ''messed up'' his learning and interfered with his wish to do well.

A PHASE OF ANALYTIC WORK
DURING ADOLESCENCE

Before Bruce reached puberty, I was puzzled by the fact that he often seemed more comfortable with his feminine identifications than with his masculine strivings. I wondered how his transvestite symptom, which had yielded only to family pressure, and his feminine identifications could protect him from castration anxiety. Material from the beginning of his adolescence helped to clarify these problems. Some interviews of this period will be presented in greater detail.

When Bruce and his brother showed signs of approaching puberty in their thirteenth year, their father talked with them about sexual development and intercourse. This discussion took place in an atmosphere of excitement and made Bruce very anxious. He avoided speaking of the talk for a while and then, when I had broached the subject, he made a drawing of a woman wearing an apron. He explained, "She's been doing the dishes and now she's painting her nails red." He thought of a TV commercial for dishwashers which contained the pun that to wash dishes was "dish-gusting." I asked Bruce, "Is it hard to let me know about the talk with your father because you found some of it worrying or disgusting?" Bruce replied that his father had said these things should not be talked about with women. I said that his father wanted to respect women's feelings but I thought he would agree to our trying to understand the worries Bruce had about sex. Bruce replied that he was confused by his father's talk; he had been most confused and worried by the discussion of menstruation. He could not remember the word at first and then recalled having felt sick a while back when he had found "something red" in the garbage. He asked his father about it and had been told not to look but to put it in the incinerator. Bruce said he knew the "something red" was blood and I replied how frightening it was to see this without being able to understand it. Bruce said he was confused by what menstruation had to do with intercourse. He also, for the first time, referred to a woman's "crotch." I suggested that it seemed especially scary to be reminded by his father how women are made differently from men.

In the following hour, Bruce expressed concern about his mother's health and spoke more about menstruation and intercourse. He then asked me whether nuns and unmarried women could menstruate; he did not think so. I said it seemed that Bruce had the worrisome idea that menstruation was like a wound, a wound which came from lovemaking. I did not yet appreciate the defensive function of Bruce's fantasy about unmarried women, that is, he could protect himself from the anxiety which knowledge of the female genitalia aroused if he could believe that unmarried women were different, not castrated. From time to time, Bruce had speculated about my life and had considered some of the advantages in living alone as an adult. The following material made it clear to me that when Bruce's feminine wishes, whether primary or defensive, became strong, he warded off castration anxiety by a specific identification, that is, with ''a woman with a penis'' (Fenichel, 1930).[5]

In one hour, Bruce complained that the coach at football had not given him enough chances to play in a football game. He then became preoccupied with his costume for a Halloween party, saying that he did not know why this was so important to him. When he had been younger he had mostly worn animal costumes. He then thought of the times he had acted in Cub Scout plays. I reminded him that then he had sometimes been chosen to play girls' parts and worn girls' costumes. He looked upset and said he did not think that he could wear a girl's costume now. I suggested that it could be hard for him to know what to wear because it was so hard to know which way he wanted to grow up. I thought that there were times when he felt very disappointed with his efforts as a boy: for instance, when he did not do as well as he had hoped to do in football he wondered if life would be better for him as a girl. To this, Bruce replied, ''Girls have it easier because no one minds them wearing boys' clothes.''

Bruce came unusually late to the next appointment and commented that nearly all of the time was gone. He was preoccupied with a woman he had seen on the way to the hour, describing her dress as "a long red and yellow one, a sari, I think." He thought that she was "a rich student who had come here from abroad." "Some of these students are very intelligent," he added. He next commented that the red of my sweater was like that of the woman's dress. I said that he was thinking of a way in which the student and I were alike, perhaps we could understand more about this. Bruce thought that I had shown intelligence, on the previous day, in what I had said about his problem. He began again to talk about his Halloween costume and spoke of his wish to go "trick or treating at rich people's homes, as they give better candy." I asked whether he was still having a thought about me. Bruce replied, "I think from your clothes and where you live you're rich and lucky, and you're smart because you learned the language here quickly." Bruce then stopped talking and sat quietly with a dreamy look in his eyes. After a while, I commented on this faraway, dreamy look and asked if he had more thoughts that he could share with me. When Bruce said he did not know, himself, what he was thinking, I reminded him of where our conversation had stopped. I said that Bruce had told of all the advantages which he imagined I had. I wondered if he had been dreaming of being like me and if he might think of me as so fortunate because of some other advantage that he thought I had.

In a following hour, Bruce asked me what I had meant by "another advantage." I said that I wanted to share with him my ideas about why he thought I was so fortunate and how this fitted with his difficulty in making up his mind about his costume. I asked him to imagine how people look to a little boy of about his brother Peter's age. At first such a little boy supposes that there are no differences between boys and girls and that everyone is made like him. When they notice a girl's body for the first time, they do not know how to understand what they see; they worry whether the little girl has been hurt and feel scared that they might be hurt in the same place. To spare themselves this worry, some boys just don't "believe their eyes and stick with their old idea that girls, too, have a penis." Bruce looked quite anxious as I spoke and, with a sudden movement, pulled a loose thread from his shirt sleeve. I said it looked as though he was remembering and feeling the old worry from the time he was about Peter's age. I thought that this worry had been so big that he "hadn't been able to believe his eyes" and had managed to go on believing that girls and women do have penises beneath their dresses. I thought that this was the real advantage that he thought I had as an unmarried woman. His debate about his Halloween costume seemed to say, "It's too hard growing up to be a man; it's too scary to be a woman; the best way out would be to be a woman with a penis." At first, Bruce said that he thought this was a crazy idea but then recalled an observation which he had made of his mother "when she seemed to have a penis."

When he was nearly 14, Bruce's reaction to Bill's check-up at the hospital for possible appendicitis threw further light on his bisexual conflict. On the day of the check-up, which had taken place on short notice, Bruce first spoke of a football game in which he had felt scared because the other team "tackled them too low." He next considered his Halloween costume and said that he would like to be one of the Three Musketeers. I asked what he knew about them, he replied, "Not much," and went on to describe what he might wear as a Musketeer: baggy trousers, his mother's blouse, because it had ruffled cuffs, and a cowboy-type hat. Bruce commented that this was the kind of costume people had worn in the old days. This reminded me of a dream which Bruce had reported two days previously and in which he was with another boy and two girls. In the dream, they had white heads, "I mean hair as they did in the time of George Washington. They were living in a wood, I think, and there was old-fashioned music." I said that in the dream, too, Bruce had been thinking of the old days and of different ways of dressing. In recalling the dream again, Bruce said that it was like a "masquerade and that the boys and girls wore

clothes that were very much alike.'' He then revealed that Bill had
been sick for a few days, throwing up, and that when he, Bruce,
had come home from school the day before, he had heard that Bill
had gone to the hospital to be checked for appendicitis. I wondered
if Bruce had not told me before about Bill's throwing up because
he was so worried about him. Bruce belittled his concern, adding
that Bill was ''okay'' and had not even had to stay overnight at the
hospital. I said that he was letting me know that if Bill had stayed
overnight then he would really have had to worry and in this way
he might be letting me know how difficult some other hospital
times had been for him.

At this point, Bruce recalled his tonsillectomy, saying that the
worst had been ''the smell of the gas, having it done when they
were asleep and wearing short gowns, instead of pajamas.'' I
wondered if there was a link between this memory of the hospital
and the dream with a masquerade in which boys' and girls' clothes
were alike. Bruce replied, ''That's not very difficult. 'Masquerade' is like doctors' masks and boys and girls wore the same
gowns in the hospital; they were short with a slit in them.'' Bruce
next remembered having been puzzled that he did not have a scar
and asked where the tonsils were; he reflected that he now knew
they were in the throat but had not known then and had thought that
they were ''down there,'' pointing to his navel; but he also remembered having had a sore throat. I said that this must have been
such a frightening experience in the hospital when he had not been
able to know the facts. I added that often a little boy worried that
the doctor would operate on his penis; I added that I thought his
memory of the hospital gowns showed us that he, too, had had the
worrisome idea that a hospital ·was a place where boys could be
made like girls. Bruce recalled having felt miserable when his
gown had ''wriggled up,'' leaving his penis uncovered. I sympa-
thized with the fact he must have felt his penis was in danger,
adding that it could be this old feeling, from that time, which
scared him about ''being tackled low'' at football. I also linked his

need to play down Bill's current symptoms and check-up with his "old hidden idea" about what could happen to a boy at the hospital.

This material próvided the link between Bruce's passive wishes and his castration anxiety. The fantasy that boys become like girls in the hospital expressed a wish and also evoked a fear of injury. It became possible now to understand the relation between defense, anxiety, and wish which was portrayed in his transvestite symptom. His defensive identification with a woman with a penis protected him from the castration anxiety caused by his passive wishes.

The reader may question at this point the relative meaningfulness of the material to Bruce and to the analyst. The analytic work presented here gave Bruce an introductory insight into his bisexual conflicts. Further working through was necessary and became possible in the context of primal scene material.[6]

SUMMARY

The material in Bruce's prepubertal phase of treatment demonstrated how he warded off feelings of loss or rivalry at the pregenital level by mechanisms of introjection and identification. His close relationship with his twin no doubt fostered these mechanisms and made individuation more difficult for Bruce. He became like mother or sister in taking over their clothes or jewelry and in this way spared himself painful feelings of abandonment and loss. In prepuberty, competitive masculine strivings at the phallic level aroused more castration anxiety than feminine ones and were dealt with by avoidance and restriction of activity.

During the adolescent phase of treatment, the structure of Bruce's transvestite symptom was clarified. In Bruce's fantasy a woman's clothes concealed a penis. By identifying with this woman, *passive wishes* could be satisfied without fear of castration.

NOTES

[1] I learned from his reaction that beginning the analysis at this time was too stressful for Bruce. It faced him with separations at home and in treatment which were too hard to master. It would have been better to postpone treatment until the New Year.

[2] Burlingham's (1950) observation of twins in the Hampstead Nurseries showed that at about ten months the twin who was not picked up or fed first by the mother or nurse "objected to being the one who was left behind. This may be the origin of the competition between the twins expressed later by the refrain 'Me too', 'Me first', 'Only me'."

[3] Bruce experienced the same feelings of worthlessness and fear of rejection in adolescence about nocturnal emissions.

[4] See Demarest and Winestine (1955), Joseph and Tabor (1961), Leonard (1961), Burlingham and Barron (1963).

[5] In his paper "The Psychology of Transvestitism," Fenichel drew attention to the transvestite's identification with the woman with a penis.

[6] Memories and reconstruction of the primal scene promoted analysis of Bruce's difficulties in spelling and reading accurately. These were connected with an inhibition of looking and registering what he had seen.

BIBLIOGRAPHY

Arlow, J.A. 1960. Fantasy systems in twins. *Psychoanalytic Quarterly* 29:175-99.

Burlingham, D.T. 1946. Twins, environmental influences on development. *Psychoanalytic Study of the Child* 2:61-75.

Burlingham, D.T., and Barron, A.T. 1963. A study of identical twins: Their analytic material compared with existing observation data on their early childhood. *Psychoanalytic Study of the Child* 18:367-423.

Demarest, E., and Winestine, M.C. 1955. The initial phase of concomitant treatment of twins. *Psychoanalytic Study of the Child* 10:336-52.

Fenichel. O. 1930. Zur Psychologie der Transvestitismus. *Internationale Zeitschrift fur Psychoanalyse* 16:21-34. Republished in *Collected papers*, First series, 1953. New York: W.W. Norton.

Freud, A. 1965. *Normality and pathology in childhood*. New York: International Universities Press.

Joseph, E.D., and Tabor, J.H. 1961. The simultaneous analysis of a pair of identical twins and the twinning reaction. *Psychoanalytic Study of the Child* 16:275-99.

Leonard, M.R. 1961. Problems in identification and ego development in twins. *Psychoanalytic Study of the Child* 16:300-20.

A Contribution to the Study of Homosexuality in Adolescence

Marjorie P. Sprince *London*

INTRODUCTION

Much has been written about the physiological changes of adolescence and the redistribution of libido that accompanies it (Deutsch, 1947). The characteristic qualities of the adolescent upheaval have been described in detail by Anna Freud (1958), Blos (1962), Geleerd (1957, 1958), Jacobson (1961), and Winnicott (1962).

One of the features of this phase of development is the transitory nature of characteristics such as excessive independence or dependency, defiance, outraged protest, delinquency, promiscuity, or homosexuality. At the time of their appearance these can be so overwhelming that they frighten both the adolescent and his environment. Indeed it is often difficult for the therapist to disentangle transitory adolescent features from true pathology. It is only when a developmental reconstruction can be made in the course of diagnosis and therapy that a clear distinction between pathology and the normal adolescent process can be attempted. Even then

This paper is based upon a paper of the same title read at a study weekend of the Association of Child Psychotherapists in March 1963 and on a publication in the *Journal of Child Psychology and Psychiatry*, vol. 5 (1964), Pergamon Press Ltd. I am indebted to the editors of this journal and to the Pergamon Press for permission to republish this paper in its present, extended form.

prognostic predictions are hazardous and must take into account not only qualitative and quantitative factors, assessment of ego strength, and so on, but the unknown influence on each individual ego of the adolescent process which may tip the balance in one direction or the other, that is to say towards homosexuality or heterosexuality. It should be borne in mind that homosexual and heterosexual strivings can be said to compete with each other throughout normal development.

This paper is written as a contribution towards the study of homosexuality in adolescence in an attempt to distinguish normal adolescent features from pathology. While I have drawn from experience with a number of cases, the paper is based upon the detailed analytic material of one boy of 16, already an overt homosexual when he entered treatment.

It is important to emphasise at the outset how my technique was guided and influenced by the severity of this boy's pathology as it gradually manifested itself in the treatment situation.

In my opinion the very rare need to introduce technical devices (such as the provision of food which I shall describe) must in itself be considered a pointer to the level of disturbance one is dealing with and a criterion of the extent of regression and possible ego damage.

BACKGROUND MATERIAL

Paul, the eldest of one sister and three brothers, had by the age of 15 changed from a 'gentle loving son' into a violent and destructive adolescent, incapable of holding down a job because of phobic anxieties. He was prone to extreme outbursts of temper with his mother, which were so severe that both doctor and Mental Welfare Officer were frequently sent for. His demanding and infantile behaviour at home resulted in his being treated like a little king and he terrorised his entire environment. He cheated the railways, stole from his place of work, and lived a life based entirely on the pleasure principle. He had no interests or sublimations. When referred for treatment at 16, he had been having a homosexual affair for over a year with George, a man seven years older than himself, but felt drawn towards boys younger than himself. His anxiety over his temper outbursts and subsequent fear of madness motivated his co-operation in treatment. He was emphatic that he did not want his homosexuality to be "taken from him" because he "loved boys so much."

The parents were well to do and overindulgent. Their marital relationship was characterised by the father's passivity, punctuated by outbursts of violence, and the mother's dominant, possessive, and overpowerful personality. Paul had slept in his parents' bedroom until the age of 11.

TREATMENT[1]

Pre-oedipal partnership between mother and son

Paul's defensive measures in treatment soon revealed his belief that any interest on my part was an attempt to overwhelm him into submission. It was his conviction that everything of his—be it friends or ego capacities—really belonged to his mother. The defensive measures he used in the transference indicated the strength of his underlying wish to merge and be one with her, but were also expressions of strivings towards independence.

In the sessions, Paul's seductive, provocative, bantering behaviour was enacted without apparent shame or embarrassment. He would play the piano with his feet, or dress up and imitate people in authority, such as Hitler or Napoleon. Often he would develop somatic symptoms, dramatically falling onto the couch complaining of stomach upsets, giddiness, and sickness. At times his exhibitionistic behaviour would go so far that he would demand that I look at a corn and bind it up as mother would. Above all he would demand food.

The following material is taken from the fifth week of treatment and highlights the conflict between the regressive pull towards pre-oedipal body contact and the wish to "merge," and the defences against this pull.

Paul started the first session by taking off his shoes and socks and massaging his corn. He sat moaning with his eyes closed, interrupting occasionally to say that he was lonely and hungry—hadn't had anything to eat for hours—and that he wanted me to tell him how to start—what to say. "Why can't he do things himself—find the words he wants?" I spoke about his need to depend upon someone stronger than himself and how this conflicted with his wish to be a powerful person in his own right. Paul replied that mother always started off the day for him by waking him and forcing him to do things. Today he hadn't gone to work because mother had overslept after a party and had left the maid to rouse him. He hadn't heard the maid, and when mother came in later he had ignored her until she tried to use force to wake him up. Then they had a row, mother threatened suicide and Paul had fallen asleep again. I reminded Paul about the recent occasions when I had spoken to him and he had appeared not to hear me, just as he hadn't heard the maid.

Paul now asked me whether I had read *The Little Prince*, an illustrated fairy story which he had brought with him. Paul pointed to the illustrations,[2] the first, of a serpent wound round the body of a "wild beast" with the beast's head in the serpent's wide open mouth. The second showed a hat and the third the outline of a hat formed by the tail of an elephant which could be seen nestling inside the hat. Paul explained that the author really understood children and he judged everyone by the way they understood his pictures. The point was whether you saw the pictures as representing a boa constrictor who had swallowed an elephant or merely saw a hat.

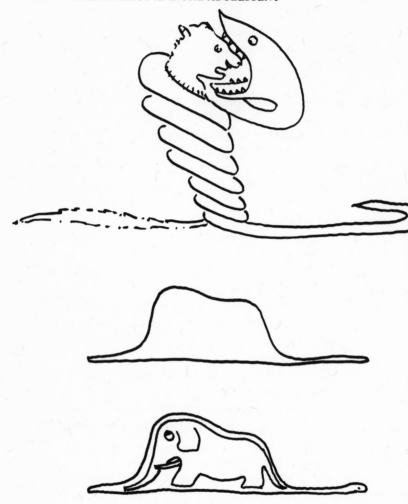

I said that Paul seemed concerned that I might not understand him and recognise the frightened wild child inside the
apparently grown-up boy. Paul went on to tell me how the
Little Prince preferred looking forward to things rather than
having the actual things themselves. It reminded him of the
film *The Blue Angel*, which described how women made men
depend upon them and then humiliated them and let them
down. We spoke of Paul's attempts with his babyish behaviour, to provoke me to control, punish, and humiliate
him. But equally he feared that I would make him dependent
upon me, unable to function unless I started him off and set
him in motion, as mother did when she waked him up and told
him what to do. At such times he felt as if he were almost a
part of mother—swallowed up by her or inside her like the
elephant in the hat. Paul said, "Like a baby before it's born."
I said that perhaps he thought that when he had been a little
baby he had never been lonely, frightened, or hungry, so part
of him longed to go back to that time.

Paul told me about his younger brother who was about to
celebrate his Bar Mitzvah. It reminded him of his own Bar
Mitzvah and how his mother had used his monetary gifts to
pay for the party he had never wanted. The party was for their
pleasure, not for his, and he was never consulted. It was taken
for granted that his money belonged to his parents. I said that
perhaps he feared that I too would treat his possessions—that
is, his thoughts and achievements, as if they were mine. Paul
became furious at this interpretation: he shouted "Shut up,"
made a gesture as if to throw a book at me, and threatened to
play the piano with his feet so that everyone would hear. He
wondered why he didn't do well at school. When he was 7,
mother had bought him a piano against father's instructions
because she wanted him to do well. Why wasn't he as intelligent as George? George wanted an intelligent boy friend. I
said that perhaps being intelligent and successful was danger-

ous because it felt like giving in—just like doing well with the piano or at school. Perhaps pleasing mother or George felt like being swallowed up by them and losing his identity. We further considered that in his work with me, Paul also feared making progress in case I treated his achievements as if they were my own.

Here Paul became excited and confused: he began to whisper that I was making him ill; he didn't know where he was; he didn't feel real. He jumped up and started to tear a book into pieces. I said that the thought of being swallowed up by me—becoming a part of me—terrified him. It made him feel as if he weren't himself, not real. At such times he had to do something destructive so that he could see that he *was* really there and not a part of someone else.

Paul thought all this might be true because he didn't want to be influenced by me and see things through my eyes as he did through mother's eyes when she persuaded him to give up his boy friends because they were scruffy. This referred to an incident he had already described when at the age of 8 his mother had succeeded in putting an end to a friendship that he had valued. This incident was now elaborated and confused with a subsequent incident, when his mother was said to have sent away a boy friend without telling Paul that he had called, and still later when she tried to eject George. Paul thought that if mother had let him have boy friends, they would have introduced him to girl friends, too.

Paul did in fact have two close childhood girl friends, but at the time of these sessions he had not remembered them. What he did remember, however, was his feeling "that in having boy friends he was taking something from mother." He went on to consider that he still had this feeling. This was probably a reversal of his own experience with his brothers who he felt had usurped his place with his mother. A later memory seemed to be relevant. Paul told me of the time when he and his parents had been travelling by car to a holiday resort. Suddenly mother had stopped the car to praise two strange boys and compare them favourably with Paul. Paul had felt "criticised, different, and hurt"; he had got out of the car and hit the boys.

Paul's intense jealousy of his two brothers was further complicated by his conviction, confirmed by his parents' statements, that mother had wanted him to be a girl. There were photos of Paul at age 3, dressed in girlish clothes and with long curly hair. Mother was said to have cried when he had his curls cut off. His sister's birth, when he was 11, seemed to have confirmed existing fantasies rather than to have initiated them. His symptoms became more acute and ultimately helped him to perpetuate his role as "little prince" in the family and thus focus his mother's entire attention on himself.

Suspicion that his central position in the family was at the cost of his masculinity and independence was uppermost in the early days of treatment. Paul complained tearfully and continuously that people treated him as the feminine partner in his relationship with George; that he didn't want to look girlish. Was his figure feminine; did he look manly; were his clothes too feminine? He enacted this dilemma over his sexual identity ceaselessly in his sessions. The following material is taken from the seventh week of treatment:

> Paul had been furious with me because I had not opened the door to him personally but had permitted the housekeeper to let him in. It now emerged that he had not been to work since mother had overslept and had sent the maid to wake him in her place. When I drew attention to the similarity of these two incidents, Paul ordered me to read aloud to him from *The Little Prince*. When I remained silent he started to weep, to beg, and then finally to become abusive. He shouted the words he had previously used about his mother—"You are

wicked, loathsome; I hate you.'' As usual he followed this by feeling sick and ill. I showed him his distress and anger when he felt that he was not the center of my or mother's life and how he had to regress to utter dependence, illness, and even girlishness to get the attention he so needed. I thought his anger and attempts to overpower me had to do with his own experiences of being overpowered in the past. Paul responded by shouting, ''Don't speak, don't speak, listen.'' He then started reading loudly and rapidly from *The Little Prince* so that for ten minutes I was effectively silenced. Ultimately, I was able to slip an interpretation between sentences: I said that not only was he having to provide for himself the story that I had refused him, but he seemed to have to do it in such a way as to overwhelm and silence me. Perhaps this was what had happened to him.

Paul could now tell me of his mother's ceaseless scenes and verbal attacks. These were particularly associated in his mind with her complaints that he wasn't the loving and affectionate boy he used to be and how she wanted to know exactly where he had been and what he would be doing. In this context he told me that he had continued to go to his mother's bed for cuddles until a year previously. We discussed Paul's vacillations between passive dependence and physically aggressive behaviour in terms of his attempts at anticipation and mastery—that by provoking, he could bring about at will the attack which he both longed for and dreaded. This reminded him of a film on television which he and his parents had recently watched together. It concerned a mother who so dominated her son that he nearly murdered her. Paul wondered if his parents had understood the implications.

Paul's fear of his phallic mother, who could arouse him to a pitch of excitement or murderous violence, brought with it a terror of loss of control and madness. It was a recurrent theme throughout treatment. The following fragment of a session comes from the phase of treatment we are now discussing:

Paul started the hour with a "ritual programme" in which he clowned an imitation of powerful or important people. This was followed by a flood of questioning and then a withdrawal into complaints and silence. When I showed him the defensive nature of this behaviour, he told me that Freud believed in horoscopes and he wanted me to tell him about Taurus: Was it a bull with a horn? Was Freud a mad old man? What was his daughter like? Did I work with her? And so on. I commented on the questions and related them to mother's questioning. Paul asked, "How does the trick of seeing through a blindfold work? You're in the same line of business." I said that he had to defend himself against me, just as he had to defend himself against mother, because I too questioned him. At times it might seem that I was in 'the same line of business,' that is to say that I too wanted to possess and control him. We could now discuss how Paul had to use every method available to defend himself against mother's "penetration." The danger was that I (mother) would get at his secrets and discover his vulnerability and thereby be able to arouse feelings in him which he felt he couldn't control. The reference to the horoscope contained the fear that no defense could succeed because destiny was already decided at birth.

Passivity: Withdrawal into sleep

As his behaviour was understood and interpreted, Paul introduced into his treatment a further characteristic of his relationship to his parents: for many weeks he gave up speaking in his sessions. For long periods Paul had refused to address his parents, since speaking to them implied "giving in." Instead, he had invented a mime language (which he called "middle language") to make his demands for food and clothes known. In this way he regressed to something akin to pre-verbal communication. The not speaking soon developed into a further regression. Paul fell asleep as soon as he sat in his chair and often remained asleep for an entire hour. At such times he appeared not to hear me when I spoke to him, or to awaken if I made a noise. At no time did I touch him physically to rouse him, but I did on occasions move about the room and open a cupboard door. In this way I nearly always managed to wake him in time to warn him of the approaching end of the session. When I succeeded in rousing him he would tearfully plead for food and drink, ask what he would do if I were not there to stop him from being angry, or protest in tears that he wanted to be a man. The tendency to sleep increased and impeded effective analytic work for a period of three months until technical devices were introduced which will be referred to later. The following material is taken from the twenty-sixth week of treatment:

Paul came to the session begging me to "start him off" and complained that his parents should have sent him to a decent school so that he would be better equipped. Mother had had a good education but didn't make use of her opportunities. He always had to be pushed, couldn't remember things, wasn't intelligent—something must be wrong with his mind. I said that he felt that he had been born "wrong" and that there was nothing that he could do about it. Paul said that he couldn't control himself. He started to close his eyes, appeared to fight against going to sleep, and remarked that he didn't like going to sleep alone at home; he got lonely. At this point, he fell asleep and remained apparently inaccessible for about thirty minutes. During this time I made interpretations about his need to shut me out, not to hear me, as he had pretended not to hear the maid, and as he wished not to hear mother when she attacked him. I also spoke about his sleeping as a defense against being angry with me.

When Paul awoke he seemed dazed and confused. I remarked that there were still ten minutes left of the session and I repeated the interpretation about his need to shut me out as he had done to the maid and would like to do with his mother. Paul protested that he wasn't affected by his mother: "She can't reach me; it's sickly, horrible." Angrily he said that he didn't want to speak about it and then added petulantly that it wasn't fair, my letting him sleep: "You don't care whether I sleep or not; you've bewitched me, got me in your power." I said that his sleeping in the hour seemed to have another purpose, that of trying to force me to wake him, touch him, and fight with him as mother did. In this way he would turn the tables on me and have *me* in his power. Paul asked why he should want to do this and then told me that he provoked the same battles with George when he stayed with him. George had to wake him repeatedly, make breakfast for him, and plead with him in an attempt to get him to work.

The next session continued with the same theme. Paul's eyes closed, but opened again when I asked if he were about to go to sleep. He said that his trouble was that he couldn't bring himself to leave George although he didn't think he loved him. He was in fact always thinking of younger boys; but what would happen to him when he was 40 if he left George? He wanted to love George and just be friends with him. He really wanted to leave George but "he can't say 'no'; he has never been able to say 'no.'" Had I really bewitched him yesterday? I must be cunning. I said that since mother, George, and I seemed so powerful he could only say "no" by shutting us out, either by sleeping or refusing to speak.

The determinants of Paul's need to sleep were many. Sleep demonstrated the passivity through which Paul warded off his intense aggression, aggression from which he protected me, while at the same time avoiding the projected retaliation he anticipated from me. Sleep also demonstrated the longed-for passive submission to his mother and must be considered in relation to his ego regression and the wish to return to the womb which has been shown as an expression of the wish to merge. The conflict between passivity and aggression which was behind Paul's extreme ambivalence could be seen in every sphere of his life.

Paul's dependence and terror of separation were so marked that gross somatic symptoms would appear before holidays or separations from his analyst. At such times he would ring me, threatening to be ill, to lose his job, or even to be promiscuous, if he could not see me. The extent of these symptoms led him to acknowledge the fact that dependence was the price he had to pay for continuing to have his mother in his power and thereby remain her sole concern.

Paul was constantly preoccupied with breaking free from his mother and leaving home. His ideas of an independent existence were totally unrealistic and revealed fantasies of luxurious living like members of the Royal Family, many of whom he insisted were homosexual. His picture of himself surrounded by velvet drapes, plush carpets, and tended by an elderly male valet revealed the extent to which he identified with his luxury-loving mother in her relationship to his father, who provided her with lovely clothes and jewellery. In the transference, he showed this identification when he used her methods of threatening illness and suicide, or demanded drugs and sedatives. His passive behaviour was characterized too by his methods of manipulation, and his pleas for hypnotism and someone to make all decisions for him.

The primary significance of the sleeping, however, was the wish to force me into bodily intimacy with him. It emerged that the major battles between mother and son were centered round oral dependency and bodily intimacy. I have described how Paul would refuse to wake up until his mother had come to rouse him personally. There would follow a sadomasochistic scene in which Paul would continue to sleep until finally she attacked him physically. The ensuing battle would continue until one or the other was hurt. Often family members and the doctor would be involved, until finally, in a state of extreme distress, Paul would remain in bed all day, thus staying away from work. The collusion among all members of the family in this situation needs no comment.

Paul's dependent behaviour in the transference, his demands for food, his aggression, and his withdrawal into sleep all indicate a regression to a narcissistic stage of development. This pre-oedipal regression is characterized by an object relationship in which the need satisfying function of the object is more important than the relationship itself, and this is fully confirmed by his fixation to the oral level.

It now emerged that one characteristic of Paul's homosexuality was the selection of older boys who would entirely take over his mother's role. Thus by demanding that George wake him up in the morning and cook for him the partnership soon followed the identical pattern of his relationship with his mother, centering round the familiar sadomasochistic rows and violent attacks, demonstrations of wounds, and dramatic reconciliations. While defending against his passive wishes by protestations of manliness and equality, Paul longed for, but feared, anal penetration. Above all he believed his love objects to be social and intellectual paragons who must become entirely dedicated to him. It had to be "as if they were one." If he possessed his love object entirely he would also possess his virtues and his penis. This repetition of an aspect of the mother relationship illustrates clearly the regression to primary identification, that is, the wish to merge with the object.

The secret guilt behind these relationships was that all Paul's thoughts and fantasies concerned not the chosen partner, but young boys whom he could love and protect. Thus the ambivalence and the conflict between active and passive wishes was once again crucial.

Paul's resistance to talking about younger boys was based upon a fear that treatment would cause him to lose interest in them. In his narcissistic fantasies he imagined comforting these lonely and frightened boys when they too made the terrible discovery of their own homosexuality. His longing to do for others what he had once longed for himself, revived memories of older women loving him protectively.

Oral and anal development

It was the need to deal with the long periods of sleep, which appeared not to be feigned and therefore left me unsure whether interpretations got through, that led me to consider whether this very infantile ego should not be handled in ways more appropriate to its stage of development. I decided that by partially satisfying Paul's oral longings, I might encourage him to a further step forward which would at least enable him to listen to my interpretations. I therefore resorted to the device of providing him with the tea which he missed at work because of his treatment. I explained that I was doing this because of his urgent need to have concrete evidence, like a small child, that I understood his empty helpless feelings. I suggested that we would continue in this way until we understood more about these feelings and why he believed that he had not the strength to help himself.

Paul used his tea, which was waiting for him when he arrived, to re-enact the oral aspect of the partnership between himself and his mother.

The following is material from the thirty-fifth week of treatment, six weeks after the "tea sessions" had been initiated. For the first week Paul had welcomed the tea and had eaten and drunk greedily. Gradually, however, he had begun to demand that I pass it to him, pour out the tea, sugar it, fetch hot water, and so on. I steadfastly refused to fulfill all such demands but instead questioned their meaning. Paul responded by depriving himself of the food he wanted while sitting complaining of hunger; he would threaten to throw the tea on the floor and would frequently leave at the end of the hour with the tea untouched.

Paul saw his tea on the table and said that he was cold, hungry, and thirsty. He complained of feeling ill and asked if he looked ill. He wanted me to tell him whether he was getting better. Who was Julius Caesar? Was he a good man? I must tell him, I must answer him at once. I said that something seemed to have upset him. Paul replied that he wouldn't tell me anything unless I answered his questions. He looked at his tea and said that he could not be bothered to reach for it, I must pass it to him. I reminded him of previous sessions when he had similarly left his tea to get cold because I had refused to sugar it. I added that Julius Caesar was a powerful emperor. Perhaps Paul thought that like a prince he could make people do anything he wanted. Paul told me to shut up, my talking made him furious, but he wasn't angry. When he got angry he would threaten to leave or throw something at me. I said that Paul's feelings were very mixed. It was true that he often felt very angry with me, but at the same time he longed to be close to me. I thought his many questions were his way of getting me to feed him as mother had fed him when he was a little child. Perhaps he had seen his little brother on mother's lap being fed and comforted in this way and wanted it for himself. Like a little child he felt unable to wait when he was hungry because he felt empty and lonely. He described it as feeling ill and that might well be how a little child felt until the mother came and fed him and made him feel well again. Paul told me to stop talking and said that he had no such recollections. He became silent and withdrawn. I said that apart from feeling angry because I wasn't feeding him with answers he also seemed frightened that I would stuff him with food (words) against his will. Paul said angrily that he couldn't hear what I was saying, that he hadn't spoken to his parents over a meal for months and he wouldn't do so now. There had been a row this morning over breakfast and he had walked out without eating; he wouldn't go home for supper tonight although his mother had rung him at work to say she expected him. I said that his question about Julius Caesar being a good man referred to himself; he felt that anyone who was so demanding and angry could not be good at the same time.

Paul demanded that I pass him his tea saying that it was my fault that it was getting cold, I would have to make him a fresh pot. In a fury he made a gesture as if to sweep the tea off the table but only hit the sugar bowl. To my question, Paul admitted that this was what had happened that morning, but the teapot and cups had broken. I said that if he could not sit on my or mother's lap and be fed, he could at least try to provoke a fight and thus achieve some body contact. We considered that the sleeping and the complaints of illness had similar meanings.

Paul was now able to tell me of the long-standing battles over meals and how he could not resist his mother's demands that he return home for all meals, because he so loved her food. He would demand food at any time and it had to be served to him by mother. Often when it arrived, however, he would sweep it aside with a complaint. What he could not understand was the uncontrollable fear and fury that overcame him at each mealtime. He dreaded every meal and could only deal with his feelings by remaining silent which incensed his parents beyond description. I said that it was frightening to feel so dependent because it made him vulnerable and therefore weak and helpless. That was why he had to hide his feelings under a show of power and strength. When it was time to leave for the weekend break, Paul became frightened and begged for a pill ''or something to make him strong.''

Once Paul was able to bring associations and memories, the acting out diminished and at his own suggestion the tea in his sessions could be abandoned.

As a small boy, Paul had been a poor eater, and his mother's preoccupation with forcing him to eat was one which he had enjoyed. Gradually the forcing and persuading him to eat had become a source of fear which he associated with being invaded, "giving in," and losing control. He began to recognise that he could control his mother by refusing food, and that in this way too he could keep out the thoughts and ideas that she pushed into him. There were also fantasies of devouring and being devoured. The need to control women orally so that they did not control him could be seen at all levels and was particularly noticeable in relation to his mother's words (and to mine). Paul's comment that he could not hear what I was saying illustrates not only his continued use of primitive defense mechanisms, but also how he sexualised words, and experienced them at this level, as phallic penetration. His longing to go back to the stage when he enjoyed being fed was always evident when he was in conflict at a further level of development, with detrimental effect upon treatment. This material illustrates the primitive mechanisms of introjection and projection characteristic of the oral phase and based upon unconscious fantasies of oral incorporation and anal ejection. These remained Paul's main mechanisms and explain his pre-oedipal identifications. Jacobson (1954) says of the infant, "Pre-oedipal identifications, magic by nature, are founded on primitive mechanisms of introjection and projection, corresponding to fusions of self and object images which disregard the realistic differences between self and object. They will find expression in illusory fantasies that the child is part of the object or can become the object by pretending to be or by behaving as if he were it" (p. 102).

The anal material implicit in much of this paper has not been dealt with specifically. It was, however, often brought in oral terms such as Paul's demand for pills and his preoccupation with being full or empty. When he felt weak he cried for strength to be "inserted." In his fantasy, the pill from me was not far removed from the idea of anal penetration by George.

Phallic development, exhibitionism, castration anxiety, masturbation

Castration anxiety is a characteristic of every analysis but it is the quantitative and qualitative factor which is significant in cases of perversion. Most psychoanalytic authors agree (Fenichel, 1946) that the homosexual is a person whose sexual pleasure is blocked by the idea of castration and that the perversion aims at denying castration so that orgasm becomes possible.

Paul's feelings of inadequacy and inferiority were evident in every aspect of his personality. Socially he considered himself an outcast, complaining that peers and aristocrats came out of the top drawer and were born with something that no one could take away, while he belonged to an inferior class and race, undistinguished, grasping, and dirty, fit only for homosexuality. Intellectually he despaired of himself; although his I.Q. was over 120, he had done badly at school and felt that all effort was futile. He saw intellectual superiority in everyone else, which was soon recognised as a displacement for his real conviction that some people were born with greater, and others with lesser, sexual capacities. He was interminably preoccupied with clothes and 'outer trappings'. His figure, the shape of his nose, the size of his hands, were constant topics of conversation.

Paul's intense exhibitionism will be illustrated in the subsequent treatment material. One aspect, however, must be emphasised. While Paul never tired of exhibiting the wounds his mother or George inflicted on him during their battles, he was even prouder of those he inflicted upon mother and George. Black eyes, scratched face, or bruised legs were brought to his sessions for admiration. He was aware that mother exhibited her wounds to others and was quick to recognize the gratification behind her complaints and demands for sympathy. On the other hand, Paul's feelings of omnipotence and guilt were so strong that he believed himself in danger of doing irreversible damage to his mother. After a battle, he would watch with terror for the arrival of a doctor or ambulance. His realistic appraisal of the danger was such that he considered the only safe measure would be for him to leave home, a measure to which his family would not agree. His exhibitionistic pride was, of course, linked with his denial of castration anxiety.

The following material comes from the thirtieth week of treatment:

Paul complained about his feet, took off his shoes and socks, and made a gesture as if to show me his corn. I said that the need to show it to me was to shock and excite me, otherwise he would have told me about it in words. Paul replaced the socks saying, "Why do I so enjoy the pain of my corn?" I said that feeling pain made him sure that the corn was really there, just as his efforts to excite or shock me by showing it to me were to convince him that he had something with which to excite me.

Paul started to clean his nails, to clown, and to play the piano. He questioned me compulsively about the irreversibility of his low intelligence: "Why was he born like that, so that nothing could alter him?" He asked anxiously why the veins on his hands stood out, was it an illness? I said that the question had a similar meaning to the worry about his corn, but that he was really concerned about quite a different part of his body. In reply, Paul took a pipe out of his pocket and put it in his mouth. He whimpered, "I do love my pipe, do you like it?" He went on to explain that he had to behave like this because he had lost all self-confidence: "It's when people think terrible things about me and George, you know." (He meant when he was taken for the feminine partner.) I said that he was worried that there was something wrong with his sexual organs and his various body complaints were to draw my attention to this worry.

Paul said angrily that some people were born with more sexual feelings than others; he never masturbated because he had no feelings. This reminded him of a man he had seen masturbating in a train some years back, and then of his childhood girl friends whom he had seen naked in the bath. He remembered chasing them with a broken violin bow and another time with a stick that broke a window.

The next day, to Paul's surprise there were further childhood memories. One recollection was of having had a sore penis and not knowing what to do; he had been terrified of showing it to father. He had always had a horror of being seen naked. From a later period, he remembered an uncle jeering at him in front of his mother and saying, "Look, we can see it, your little penis."

I said that when Paul had seen his childhood girl friends in the bath this may have shocked him into realizing that girls weren't made the same as boys. Perhaps he had thought that all children were born the same and that these girls had lost their penises by doing something to them. If this could happen to a girl, he believed it could happen to him, too.

Paul said he could remember a boy cousin wanting to touch Paul's penis but not allowing Paul to touch his. I said that this must have confirmed his idea that touching was dangerous but that it did seem that when he had played these games he had exciting feelings in his penis so that it "stood up" like the veins in his hands. But the little Paul had loved his penis so much that he had been terrified of losing it, or damaging it, so that he couldn't let himself have these feelings in case he was tempted to play with it. Thus he had transferred these feelings to other parts of his body where they could be enjoyed without danger. I said, too, that he was equally frightened of the doctor or father discovering his secret in case they punished him by taking his penis away from him.

Paul now told me that he was circumcised and how this had made him feel different from all the other boys at school. At age 9, he and his boy cousin had invented a game called "nasal interludes" in which they would visit public toilets to examine other boys' genitals and compare them with their own. The title of the game clearly indicates the mechanism of displacement upwards.

While relating these memories, Paul suddenly jumped from his chair terrified that his leg had got stiff: "It wasn't pins and needles, what should he do?" We could now openly discuss how erections mobilised his castration fears and how he had to touch his penis repeatedly to make sure that it was still there and undamaged. This led to material surrounding his fear, and wish, that he might change into a girl.

Paul's castration panic was frequently expressed in somatic form. His stealing increased markedly at this stage, and he would exhibit spoils to me, bringing in phallic objects such as an umbrella, fountain pen, and key ring. We were thus able to understand the stealing as a symbolic reassurance that he could obtain an adequate penis through his own efforts. The correctness of this interpretation was confirmed by the diminution of the symptom until it disappeared entirely.

Masturbation was Paul's only real sexual pleasure and one which he felt nothing else could replace. Mutual sex play with boys of his own age had appeared in latency. Then, as later, Paul maintained that it was loneliness that drove him to find a sexual partner. In mutual masturbation, he could play both active and passive roles, which is why he dreaded abandoning it.

The swing between pre-oedipal and oedipal strivings

It is perhaps a confusing characteristic of work with adolescent homosexuals that the quantity of oedipal material leads one to assume (at times mistakenly) that these boys have solved their oedipal conflict successfully and are firmly established at the phallic level. It is a fact, however, that physiological development during puberty gives rise to increased sexual fantasies and attempts at adjustment which in some cases are misleading (Kut-Rosenfeld and Sprince, 1963). In common with borderline children, it seems that the phallic material can have something of an 'as if' quality, and is characterised by a fluid interchange between oedipal and pre-oedipal strivings. In such cases there is at best an unstable primacy of phallic development which gives way to pre-oedipal features indicating that phase dominance has not been achieved (Kut-Rosenfeld and Sprince, 1963).

Paul's material, both in the transference and in recollections, indicated what might be described as a 'flirtation' with the oedipal phase. The characteristic feature was the conflict between his oedipal strivings and the regressive pull to pre-oedipal satisfactions in which he could re-establish a close body tie to his mother. Paul tried repeatedly to separate his parents and would complain of father to mother and hint to father of mother's unfaithfulness. This mother's seductive behaviour, her manner of feigning illness to get Paul's sympathy and physical affection, her dramatic scenes in which she would plead, weep, and accuse Paul of killing her, her confidences about past lovers, all stimulated him sexually. He considered his mother's behaviour to be that of a prostitute and often called me a prostitute, explaining affectionately that "paying for treatment was like paying for sex." Threats of aggression towards his mother and myself expressed his belief that force and violence were masculine attributes proving him capable of being a lover, himself. He had once told his mother that he would never marry any other girl but her.

Paul had always been convinced that his homosexual problem

had to do with his close intimacy with his mother's body, and his fear that insight into this fact would bring about a cure and deprive him of gratification suggested to both of us that he was not entirely committed to homosexuality, or that at least there was still some conflict.

The following material from the forty-first week of treatment illustrates how fleeting heterosexual interest gave way to pre-oedipal strivings and homosexual wishes. The session followed material in which Paul told me how, at age 11, he had shared his mother's bed and had examined her body while talking intimately to her.

Paul saw me note the change of time for his next appoint-ment in my diary. He asked if it were a private diary, whether I showed it to my husband and whether I would show it to him. His anger at my refusal was discussed in connection with his jealousy of his father's rights to see his mother's genitals and equally of his mother's inability to set limits with Paul.

Paul now told me how for years it had been his custom to sit with his mother while she bathed, promising never to tell his father, a secret he had not betrayed. We discussed how this close proximity to mother had excited him to the point of violence (because of the danger of merging) and also had made him feel guilty towards his father. I said that with the adolescent heightening of sexual feeling, it was understand-able that his mother's behaviour and demands had become increasingly frightening to him. Paul said that I made him think things which weren't true; that it was natural for a boy of 15 to see his mother naked; that he had no feelings at all and never had. I said that we were beginning to understand that he feared having too many strong feelings, not too few.

This made Paul remember a funny television film of a boy

who had hidden himself under a bed while two elephants were having sexual intercourse. The bed had bumped up and down and the boy had been frightened lest he be squashed. Paul had often shared his parents' bed but he was sure that he had never seen them in the act of coitus.[3] He laughed uproariously and excitedly about the film and went on to describe vividly the terrible panics he had experienced as a child when his parents had fought with each other. At such times he would scream at them and hit them in an attempt to stop them from killing each other. It was usually mother who scratched father.

I said that Paul's idea of sexual intercourse was of a terrible battle in which the woman first seduced and then damaged the man. His investigations of his mother had to do with his conviction that she either had a penis of her own or wished to take Paul's or his father's. We discussed how terrifying this was to Paul who feared that his love for his mother might result in his losing all he valued. No wonder he had to protect himself with all means possible.

Paul arrived next day, petulant, hungry, and helpless. He complained that the light was too bright for his eyes and that modern gadgets were no good. He feared that I was angry with him and then wanted me to fix a chain around his neck, saying that he couldn't really bear a woman to touch him: "They've got nothing to lose." He said he wanted to sleep and closed his eyes, opening them a few minutes later to tell me about a man-eating spider he had seen at the zoo, where he had been with George. I said that sleep was a protection against the spider therapist who he felt might swallow up not only his penis but the whole of him. Since we knew that sleep provoked mother to both cuddle and attack him, there was a part of Paul that wanted to be swallowed up and taken inside her. Paul said, "Like the elephant in the hat." I said that the elephant was characterised by his penis-like nose and

Paul had picked on him to show me how the penis stood for the whole of him.

Paul told me of a film in which a homosexual man was wanted by the police for running a house where homosexual boys were brought together. The mother of one of the boys bribed a maid to undress in front of her son "to bring him back to heterosexuality." But the mother was finally punished by the police for turning the maid into a prostitute. I said that Paul believed that both mother and I were determined to tempt him back to heterosexuality for our own purposes, to deprive him of his organ and have it for ourselves. Thus, when he was seductive or provoked quarrels with his mother or myself, it was not only because he longed for intimacy and excitement, but to prove that he could protect his valued possession.

Paul told me of a boy of 13 whom he would like to make love to and then started to play with his tie, imagining that it was a puppet, a cobra with poisonous teeth. Suddenly, putting his hand over his penis protectively, he said he could not speak of such things to a woman. When I commented upon the way he was protecting his organ he replied without hesitation, "You've got your hand on your penis too." I reminded Paul of his wish and fear of merging (depicted by the elephant inside the hat) and of the picture of the boa constrictor wrapped round the body of a beast whose head it was about to swallow. I said that Paul wished to love a younger boy in the way he really wanted myself or mother to love him. In this way his homosexuality protected him from the man-eating spider or the toothlike vagina which he feared would swallow up his penis-nose which represented himself. But equally he feared the penetrating penis which he believed I and his mother possessed. The boa constrictor with its huge mouth was a composite of both.

Discussion of this fantasy which had oral and anal ramifica-tions, enabled Paul to understand some of the motives behind his passivity and violence in terms of the struggle around merging with his mother and the dread of losing his feeling of 'selfness'. The story of the film about the mother who persuaded the maid to save her son from homosexuality referred to an overdetermined experience at age 15 which had to be evaluated in the light of our knowledge of Paul's flight from heterosexuality. It added to the terror of merging and loss of separateness, the fears aroused at the sight of the castrated female body, and it demonstrates Paul's solution. Paul had wanted to go out one night with his parents, and when refused, had made a suicidal gesture. He had been found and comforted by a maid of 18 with whom he initiated sexual inter-course and achieved orgasm which he did not enjoy. He had subsequently invited some boys to the house, promising them the maid, but had seduced them himself. This had been his first overt homosexual experience.

Paul's relationship to his father

Paul desperately resented his helplessness and feelings of in-adequacy. For many years he had countered it with his 'Little Prince' fantasy. Like the little prince in the fairy tale, Paul com-pensated for his feelings of inadequacy and dependence by ruling the family. His fear was of identification with the king, a castrated father who, in the fairy story as in Paul's own life, was depicted as a pathetically helpless figure of fun who could only pretend to rule. But Paul did not really consider his father to be a figure of fun and this was probably denial or reversal. In fact the father's outburst of temper at times matched Paul's own in intensity and certainly terrified him. Outbursts of displeasure were expressed by physical attacks after which the father might burst into tears and plead with his son to love him again "and be nice to him." Such scenes would be followed by attempts at emotional reconciliation, accompanied by presents and bribes which Paul found both tempting and repugnant. It was characteristic of Paul's home life that both parents competed for his favours and that they viewed treatment as a similar attempt on my part.

In one area Paul admired his father: he respected and envied his social position. He identified with him, however, not in his working role but in his weaknesses, in his attitude to his wealth, in his suspected minor dishonesties, and in his outbursts of violence.

There was evidence of a disturbance in the father's relationship to his son. The material indicated the probability of unconscious homosexual problems in the father, who had never been able to tolerate a separation from the son for longer than a few hours at a time, and who would then ring him wherever he was and beg him to return.

Paul's awareness of his father's role in his life became clearer in the latter part of his treatment and was introduced in connection with his comments about older homosexual men ("queens" in homosexual jargon) who were interested in him. His longing for gifts of clothes and finery from his father was accompanied by bitter complaints that father never noticed him in the way he noticed mother. Paul began to recognise his identification with his mother as having significance in relation to his father.

The subsequent material comes from the sixtieth week of treatment. Paul was now using the couch and his sessions followed the course of a classical analysis.

We were discussing a recent battle with father about whether Paul should work with him in his firm with a view to becoming a partner. Paul told me that the bridge of his nose had been hurt and asked whether the swelling would go down. When I likened this to anxiety about erections, Paul asked me what I would do with a violent patient. I said that it seemed that he was tempting me into a battle as he so often tempted father, so that he could have an erection. Paul remembered the wolf (in the Little Prince story) who longed to be tamed but feared becoming dependent upon his tamer. This reminded him of something he had never told me: that at the age of 11 he had enjoyed beating dogs and small boys at school. He asked whether this was relevant. I said that one of his mechanisms was to do to others what he longed to have done to himself. Paul thought that the longing to be beaten went back to his early childhood and he remembered an occasion when he was 4 years old and father had hit him, Paul had masturbated again and again until he had become breathless and panic-stricken. He had called his mother but had refused to let her fetch a doctor in case the origin of his condition was discovered.

He now told me that for many years he had been unable to be alone in a room with his father or to speak civilly to him. He dreaded his father's expressions of pleasure when seeing him and responded by sullen rudeness. I said that Paul feared that his father would sense his sexual longings and would reciprocate.

In this context Paul told me of a book about two boys who had become sexual murderers. He asked whether I had read Nietzsche and told me of Nietzsche's "mad world in which the very intelligent are above the law." I said that perhaps one reason for Paul's need to prove that he was not intelligent was to reassure himself that he was in no danger of joining this mad world in which there would be no obligations or help to control his impulses. Paul said that treatment had shown him that "you lose touch with reality if you try to live like that." In *The Little Prince*, the king only pretended to have authority: he would strut about "ordering people to do the very things they wanted to do anyway." He asked what a despot was; he thought he was truly a despot because a real king recognised duties and obligations.

I said that in his childhood it had been Paul, the little

prince, who had made the laws and father who had submitted
to them. Then, and until very recently, he had recognised no
duties or obligations. But this had been very frightening to
him because he had felt there was no one who could help him
to develop control and master his impulses. We discussed
how a child develops this capacity by taking in parental
standards, and how difficult this had been for him. Paul
asked, ''Is father really weak? Have I more personality than
he?'' And then, ''Who has the greater power, a king or a
queen?''

Paul's gradual willingness to accept the limits imposed upon
him by the treatment situation, and his increased attitude of responsibility and control, led to the recognition of his wish for a
father with whom he could identify. At this stage in treatment his
aggression often gave way to depression.

The father reacted to Paul's growing insight and attempts to free
himself from his own infantile wishes and behaviour with acute
anxiety. He responded to the threatened ''loss'' by promises of
extravagant gifts and offers of luxurious holidays. As these bribes
became ever more tempting, an accompanying deterioration was
observable in Paul's behaviour. His demandingness increased, his
terror of being alone with his father returned, and once again he
became reluctant to work. Gradually the provocative rows and
violent sado-masochistic scenes so familiar with his mother and
boy friends were re-enacted with the father, but with an additional
elaboration. Far from setting limits or making demands on Paul,
each new outburst of aggression or irresponsible behaviour was
met with a reward of increasing value.

This final illustration comes from the eighty-first week of treatment. Paul was now working in his father's firm. He had abandoned his long-term alliance with George in favour of short-lived
relationships with boys of his own age or younger.

*   *   *

Paul told me about a young boy he had recently met and whom he liked. What worried him about Bob was his feeling that if he were nice to him, Bob would want him only for what he could get out of him. He felt this about all the young boys he liked so he could never trust them. I reminded him how father always asked Paul "to be nice to him" after a row and how he bribed him with gifts and money. It made Paul feel that he was nice to father only for what he could get in return; that, in fact, his relations to most people, including myself, depended upon their ability to satisfy his needs. Paul agreed that while he protested to me that father shouldn't give in to him, he demanded these gifts unceasingly. I was the only person who dared to refuse him and that made him feel safe.

I said that this showed us how far back his difficulties had started, at a time when he was so small that the people who satisfied his needs were the only ones who mattered. Paul now told me that a few days previously he had arrived late at the office to find a message asking him to go to father's room. He had gone in a state of terror, expecting to be attacked, but father had offered him the office car—father's old one—to enable him to get to work punctually. Paul had refused "because the office car is not as good as father's new one and because he wanted a coupé of his own." His father had thereupon given him an open check.

Paul asked what he should do. He knew that father shouldn't have given it to him and that he shouldn't have taken it. He hadn't earned the money. But he couldn't give it up. Why couldn't he use the office car? He'd always liked driving it before; he'd felt like a king in it.

I said that while on the one hand his refusal had to do with his wish for a battle with father, it was also an attempt to test father out and see if he would at last exert authority and set limits. But father had merely "ordered him to do the very thing he wanted to do anyway."

For many days the issue of the car was discussed, with Paul begging me simultaneously to tell him what to do and to sanction his buying the car. I said that perhaps the real point was that if he accepted father's old car he would feel more like his father and would have to take on some of the qualities which he respected in him: the obligations and responsibilities. This frightened him because it meant giving up his role as the powerful little prince. Paul said that if he bought the car, he would be letting his father buy him in the way he felt that he tried to buy younger boys, that it was the same as buying treatment or sex; ''but you only bought a prostitute's body, not her soul.'' I said that to have a car of his own which father bought him in this way, meant for Paul that he was allowing himself to be treated as a prostitute; namely, a woman like his mother or myself. It was so tempting for him because part of him still wanted father to notice him in the way he noticed mother.

I reminded Paul how, during his friendship with George, who had represented his mother, Paul had been tortured with forbidden thoughts about loving younger boys as he wanted mother to love him. Now we could see that these wishes also referred to the way he longed to be loved as a woman by his father. Paul confirmed this dilemma by telling me a story he had recently read. It concerned a 48-year-old woman—the age of his mother—who had married a 19-year-old boy and then had shot him for having a homosexual liaison.

When some days later, Paul arrived at treatment with a brand new coupé car, he had to keep his eye on the window, ''In case someone put their hand in it and meddled with it.'' ''It's an open hole, a temptation,'' he said.

To have a car of his own implied for Paul an identification with the passive seductive mother, it enhanced his femininity, and it accentuated his anxiety. While driving father's car or imagining he possessed an identical one, Paul could temporarily identify with him, thereby controlling his own and his father's homosexual urges while at the same time taking over some of his father's masculine features.

We now understood that the real threat to Paul was the temptation to accept the very gifts and luxuries that he demanded. In his own words, the acceptance of a car implied that he was allowing his father to buy him body and soul, as his mother had done with food. This reflected the conflict behind the underlying wish to merge with his father as we have seen in his other relationships, including his relationship to me in the transference. His intransigent behaviour represented his protest and fight against this wish: even if he sold his body, his soul remained his own.

DISCUSSION

The first version of this paper was published in 1964. Then, in my attempts to evaluate Paul's material I referred to many authors. These included Freud (1928), Anna Freud (1952, 1958), Gillespie (1952), Geleerd (1957, 1958), Greenacre (1952, 1955, 1960), Jacobson (1954, 1961), Nunberg (1938), Bychowski (1945, 1954, 1956, 1961). The studies of the latter on homosexuality and ego regression have been of especial interest to me.

At the time of rewriting for the present publication, Charles W. Socarides has just published his ''Theory of Aetiology in Male Homosexuality'' (1968). Much of his paper has considerable relevance to this study. While leaving my discussion much as it was in my former publication, since it deals primarily with assessment of adolescent homosexuality, I would like here to quote from Socarides' paper. Socarides sees obligatory male homosexuality as deriving from conflicts related to the earliest period of life. According to his observations:

• The preoedipal homosexual has been unable to pass successfully through the symbiotic and separation-individuation phases of early childhood. As a result of this maturational (psychological) developmental failure there are severe ego deficits. Homosexuality serves the repression of a pivotal nuclear complex: the drive to regress to a preoedipal fixation in which there is a desire for and dread of merging with the mother in order to re-instate the primitive mother-child unity (p. 33).

In the patient described by Socarides, homosexuality (1) re-assured against ego dissolution; (2) was a substitute for a reunion with the mother; (3) allowed for the expression, alleviation, and discharge of severe aggression aroused by the imperative need to merge.

It is primarily on the question of ego regression that I shall concentrate here, and the characteristic features of homosexuality will be referred to only insofar as they throw light on the question of ego disturbance and enable us to differentiate between adolescent and homosexual characteristics. It seems almost certain that while some homosexuals combine intense homosexual activity with a well-integrated and purposeful life, there are those like Paul, at the other end of the scale, who know no sublimations and whose homosexual activities pursue momentary gratification as their only aim. These are the homosexuals whose personalities are characterised by extreme persistance of infantile attitudes and narcissistic features, accompanied by magical ideas of omnipotence of thought.

If we examine the factors which are likely to have influenced Paul's development towards homosexuality, our first consideration must be the very early oral fixation linked to an overwhelming and dominant mother who was, in turn, aggressively possessive and clingingly seductive. The father was a man whose inherent passivity was interrupted at intervals by outbursts of violence. A man with latent homosexual problems of his own, he must have been both a disappointment as a model for masculine identification as well as a seductive and frightening person.

We have been able to observe the intense ambivalence to both these parents and the fact that all Paul's object relations were characterised by alternation between states of negativism and complete submission. We have also seen how he maintained object relations at the most primitive levels of oral incorporation and oral destruction. It can be recognized too that the introjected parent images seemed to be in conflict within the ego.

Bychowski (1956), speaking of this primitive ambivalence as characteristic of the homosexual, describes how its erotic component is passively anaclitic in its aims, while the aggressive component remains primitively destructive at an oral level. He further describes how the introjection of the love objects, thus invested with this very early ambivalence, leads to the development of an ego permeated with the weakness of the structure split into isolated segments.

The concept of a split in the ego was already formulated by Freud (1928) in connection with fetishism. As will be remembered, his hypothesis was that a section of the ego is split off from the rest, so that while one part maintains a correct view of reality another part denies and distorts it. This concept of an ego, part of which remains regressed in this way, would appear to explain why the homosexual shows so many psychotic features, and also why adolescent features, although present, appear only as part of the personality and have an "as if" quality. This partial ego regression, which is the immature ego's defense against pre-oedipal as well as oedipal conflicts, also explains the pregenital elements in homosexuality and why there is such difficulty in seeing the sexual partner as a whole person. It is as if one part of the ego develops or attempts to develop normally and almost independently, while the other section remains isolated and regressed.

Nunberg (1938) thinks the homosexual may be halfway between the neurotic and the psychotic, while Bychowski (1956, 1961) describes the deep affinities between homosexuals and the whole schizophrenic group. He considers them to have in general a similar psychic structure, and in particular to share many infantile qualities in libidinal organisation as well as destructive primitive features within the ego.

These statements have confirmed my conviction that some of the characteristics that appeared in Paul's material were familiar to me from observations a group of us had made in studying borderline features in near psychotic children and adolescents.[4] In particular I had noticed that Paul's ego boundaries seemed blurred so that at times he seemed unsure whether he was himself or could be someone else (as when he felt that everything of his belonged to his mother). Fleeting identifications were ominously present and the wish for (and defense against) temporary fusion with another person was clearly evident. Paul's attempts to imitate the love object with the aim of taking over that person's attributes, thereby becoming that person, have been illustrated in the material.

Such attempts to merge with the object belong to a level of early infantile development before any real object love exists, and are related to the hungry infant's longing for oral gratification and subsequent fantasies of oral incorporation (Jacobson, 1954). This longing is the origin of the first primitive types of identifications which are achieved by temporary fusions of self and object. According to Jacobson (1954), the process of refusion of self and object images in the infant is accompanied by a temporary weakening of perceptive functions, a point to be borne in mind in connection with Paul's material. These attempts at refusion of self and object mark the onset of ego formation and are the forerunners of true ego identifications, just as early reaction formations are the precursors of superego formation.

Jacobson (1954) describes the period between merging and true identification as one of constant cathectic shifts—libido and aggression turn from the object to the self, or from one object to another, and all undergo temporary fusions. These cathected processes will, she says, be reflected in introjective and projective mechanisms based on the child's unconscious fantasies of oral incorporation and anal ejection of the love object. At this stage, the child will display clinging attitudes alternating with temporary grandiose ideas of magical participation in the parents' omnipotence. There will be erratic vacillations between helpless dependency and active aggressive strivings for independence or control over the love objects. According to Lewin (1950), these attitudes go back to the two phases of oral gratification: first, when the child aggressively gets hold of the breast and drinks from it; the second, when he relaxes, becomes passive, and finally goes to sleep. With very slight variations, all this could have been written with reference to Paul at the age of 18.

This period of cathectic shifts is associated with the development of self and object images. This will be impeded if the parents' own unconscious narcissistic needs impel them to view their child as an extension of themselves. Paul's transference to me reflected his difficulties in establishing a sense of separateness. Furthermore, this process must be viewed in the context of the child's earliest experiences of safety, reliability, and predictability. This has repercussions in the widest sense on the development of self-esteem. Constant experiences of disappointment will influence not only expectations, but also the self image. The whole process profoundly influences the development of stable internalizations and therefore ego and superego formation.

Paul failed to make true ego and adequate superego identifications, and here one enters into an area where it is difficult to disentangle transitory adolescent features from homosexual characteristics. This applies to many characteristics which the homosexual and the adolescent appear to share in common, such as qualities of defiance, outraged protest, delinquency, on the one hand, and dependency on the other. Anna Freud (1958) speaks of those adolescent passionate and evanescent love fixations which are not object relations at all in the adult sense. She says they are identifications of the most primitive kind such as we meet in our study of early infantile development before any object love exists. The homosexual shares with the adolescent this tendency to fickleness which is based on a loss of personality in consequence of a change in identification.

It is necessary to evaluate these and other adolescent features in relation to developmental factors, their depth, quality, and persistence, if one is to distinguish between developmental characteristics and pathology. The point here is that in many areas, and especially that of object relationships, there are *transitory* characteristics in the adolescent which many homosexuals possess as *permanent* traits.

I have stressed the extent and depth of ego damage in this case. It follows that the earlier treatment could have been started, the better the chance of ego support and modification. Even with much earlier treatment to side with the ego against the regressive pull of the parents, difficulties would have been immense. This does not mean that in such cases modification at a later stage, and even a degree of reversibility, should be excluded as a possibility, but rather that early and deep ego damage constitutes a limiting factor in itself which must be considered in addition to the parents' pathological pull. In Paul's transference there were indications of a capacity for ego modification. We have, however, to consider whether they were based upon a forward developmental move, that is to say the possible achievement of a true identification, or whether these changes were based upon the use of the therapist as an auxiliary (borrowed) ego. (Des Lauriers, 1962).

I believe that the decisive factor in pathological homosexuality is the extent to which the ego regresses temporarily to its earliest origins, as illustrated in Paul's case. If and when reality continues to press its claims, however, unsatisfied longings become helpful to treatment. Adolescence, with its physiological upheaval which brings about instinctual chaos and unrest, increases the anxiety and disturbs the apathy. Thus adolescence with all its disadvantages for treatment also allies itself at times with therapeutic aims. It is in adolescence, when at least part of the homosexual ego is motivated by renewed attempts to sever the object tie, that passive surrender and all it implies becomes all the more terrifying. What Anna Freud (1952) said about the homosexual has, I believe, even additional validity for the adolescent homosexual:

- This fear of passivity is capable of a deeper non-sexual explanation. The passive surrender to the love object may signify a return from object love proper to its forerunner in the emotional development of the infant, i.e., primary identification with the love object. This regressive step implies a threat to the intactness of the ego, a loss of personal characteristics which are merged with the characteristics of the love object. The individual fears this regression in terms of dissolution of the personality, loss of sanity, and so on, and defends himself by a complete rejection of all objects. This assumption is confirmed by clinical examples of patients who show an alternation between states of negativism and states of complete emotional surrender to an object (p. 265).

SUMMARY

The analytic material of an overt adolescent homosexual is examined with a view to distinguishing transitory adolescent homosexual features from the permanent character traits of homosexual pathology. The factors likely to be decisive in the development of homosexuality are considered. The significance of early object relations upon the development of the ego structure is examined and affinities to the borderline psychotic ego are described, especially in relation to blurred ego boundaries and the wish to merge with the object. The disturbance is traced back to its very early origins and is understood in terms of failure to make true and adequate ego and superego identifications. It is emphasised that while the extent of ego regression appears decisive, the final outcome is difficult to predict because qualitative and quantitative factors together with the unknown influence of the adolescent process may finally tip the balance in one direction or the other. The adolescent process with its physiological upheavals bringing about increased anxiety, unsatisfied longings, and the urge towards severing the object tie is at times seen to ally itself effectively with therapeutic aims.

NOTES

[1]The present publication was prepared at Dr. Geleerd's suggestion some time before her death. Since it is a faithful representation of my technique at the time, I have not altered it substantially. In handling a similar case today I would undoubtedly concentrate more on the interference in narcissism and the painful affects associated with low self-esteem such as feelings of shame, humiliation, hopelessness.

[2]From THE LITTLE PRINCE by Antonione de Saint-Exupery, copyright, 1943 by Harcourt Brace Jovanovich, Inc., renewed 1971 by Consuelo de Saint-Exupery. Reproduced by permission of the publishers.

[3]This is an experience which is almost always repressed and the memory rarely recovered in consciousness.

[4]The group for the Study of Borderline Children at the Hampstead Child Therapy Clinic. Members of this group included Agnes Bene, Rose Edgcumbe, Dr. Fahmy, Sylvia Ini, Maria Kawenoka, Hanna Kennedy, Sara Kurt-Rosenfeld, Lily Weitzner, and the author.

BIBLIOGRAPHY

Blos, Peter. 1962. *On adolescence*. New York: Free Press of Glencoe.

Beres, D. 1956. Ego deviation and the concept of schizophrenia. *Psychoanalytic Study of the Child* 11:164-235.

Bychowski, G. 1945. The ego of homosexuals. *International Journal of Psycho-Analysis* 26:2-4.

———. 1954. The structure of homosexual acting out. *Psychoanalytic Quarterly* 23:48-61.

———. 1956. The ego and the introjects: The structure of male homosexuality. *Psychoanalytic Quarterly* 25:11-36.

———. 1961. The ego and the object of the homosexual. *International Journal of Psycho-Analysis* 42:255-59.

Des Lauriers, A.M. 1962. *The experience of reality in childhood schizophrenia*. London: Tavistock Publications.

Deutsch, H. 1947. *The psychology of women*. London: Research Books.

Eissler, K. R. 1958. Notes on problems of technique in the psychoanalytic trestment of adolescents: With some remarks on perversions. *Psychoanalytic Study of the Child* 13:223-54.

Fenichel, O. 1946. *The psychoanalytic theory of neurosis* London: Kegan Paul.

Freud, A. 1952. A connection between states of negativism and emotional surrender. *International Journal of Psycho-Analysis* 33:263-72.

———. 1958. Adolescence. *Psychoanalytic Study of the Child* 13:255-78.

Freud, S. 1928. Fetishism. *International Journal of Psycho-Analysis* 9:161-66.

Geleerd, E. 1957. Some aspects of analytic technique in adolescents. *Psychoanalytic Study of the Child* 12:263-383.

———. 1958. Borderline states in childhood and adolescence. *Psychoanalytic Study of the Child* 13:279-95.

———. 1961. Some aspects of ego vicissitudes in adolescence. *Journal of the American Psychoanalytic Association* 9:394-405.

Gillespie, W. H. 1952. Notes on the analysis of sexual perversions. *International Journal of Psycho-Analysis* 33:397-402.

Greenacre, P. 1952. Pregenital patterning. *International Journal of Psycho-Analysis* 33:410-15.

————. 1955. Further considerations on fetishism. *Psychoanalytic Study of the Child* 10:187-94.

————. 1960. Regression and fixation: Consideration concerning the development of the ego. *Journal of the American Psychoanalytic Association* 8:703-23.

Jacobson, E. 1954. The self and the object world: Vicissitudes of the infantile cathexis and their influence on ideational and affective development. *Psychoanalytic Study of the Child* 9:75-127.

————. 1961. Adolescent moods and the remodelling of psychic structures in adolescence. *Psychoanalytic Study of the Child* 16:164-83.

Kut-Rosenfeld, S., and Sprince, M. P. 1963. An attempt to formulate the meaning of the concept "borderline." *Psychoanalytic Study of the Child* 18:603-35.

Lampl-De-Groot, J. 1962. On adolescence. *Psychoanalytic Study of the Child* 15:95-103.

Lewin, B. D. 1950. *The psychoanalysis of elation*. New York: W. W. Norton.

Nunberg, H. 1938. Homosexuality, magic and aggression. *International Journal of Psycho-Analysis* 19:1-16.

Socarides, Charles W. 1968. A theory of aetiology in male homosexuality. *International Journal of Psycho-Analysis* 49:27-37.

Winnicott, D. W. 1962. Adolescence. *New Era* 43:145-51.

Mourning Accomplished by Way of the Transference

Marie E. McCann   *Cleveland*

In *Mourning and Melancholia* (1917), Freud asks the question, "In what, now, does the work which mourning performs consist?" and then proceeds with his answer:

- I do not think there is anything far fetched in presenting it in the following way. Reality testing has shown that the loved object no longer exists and it proceeds to demand that all libido shall be withdrawn from its attachments to that object. This demand arouses understandable opposition—it is a matter of general observation that people never willingly abandon a libidinal position, not even, indeed, when a substitute is already beckoning to them. This opposition can be so intense that a turning away from reality takes place and a clinging to the object through the medium of hallucinatory wishful psychosis. Normally, respect for reality gains the day. Nevertheless its orders cannot be obeyed at once. They are carried out bit by bit, at great expense of time and cathectic energy, and in the meantime the existence of the lost object is psychically prolonged.

I would like to express my appreciation to Mrs. Erna Furman, Assistant Clinical Professor, Department of Psychiatry, Case Western Reserve University Medical School, for her helpful suggestions. My thanks are also due to Dr. H. A. Scali, Director of Children's Aid Society, Cleveland, Ohio, and to the late Dr. James F. Berwald, formerly Medical Director of Children's Aid Society.

Each single one of the memories and expectations in which the libido is bound to the object is brought up and hypercathected and detachment of the libido is accomplished in respect to it (pp. 244-245).

I shall attempt to show in the analysis of Geraldine how mourning the death of her mother was made possible via the transference. Geraldine was 11 years 8 months of age when I first met her, and it had been three years and eight months since the death of her mother. She was a child who had not been capable of mourning her mother's death, which had occurred just one week before her eighth birthday. Geraldine had had the developmental readiness for mourning in that she had entered latency at the time of her loss of her mother but she had lacked several other factors essential to the accomplishment of mourning (R. Furman, 1964). That is, she had not been prepared for her mother's death in that she had never been helped to understand the realities of the terminal illness; she had lacked the assurance that her needs would be met after her mother's death; and her environment had failed to offer her any of the support necessary to enable a child to mourn.

During her mother's terminal illness and following her death, Geraldine had utilized the defense of denial of all affects and in action, by being good instead of bad. Eleven months before Geraldine had begun treatment, she had developed amnesia, and repression had blotted out not only the associated affects but also the actual reality of her mother's terminal illness and death, and her own life in the two years and nine months subsequent to the loss of her mother. Geraldine began analysis with no real memory of her mother's death, thus eliminating reality testing by which memories are assigned to the past. Her analysis continued for six and one-half years and ended when she was a little over 18 years of age, a week after her graduation from high school.

From the analytic work which extended from pre-puberty into late adolescence, I have selected the work related to the analysis of defenses which had prevented her mourning; the shifting and lifting of mechanisms; and the working through of the relationship with her mother, with facilitation of her mourning, via the transference. This thread is the focal aspect of her analysis and weaves throughout the entire period of her treatment.

PERTINENT HISTORY

Geraldine was an only child. She had a half-brother, seventeen years older than herself, and a half-sister, fourteen years her senior. The half-siblings were the children of the mother's first marriage. The mother married a second time and separated but had not yet obtained a divorce from her second husband when she began her relationship with Geraldine's father and when Geraldine was conceived. Actually, owing to further delays in obtaining the divorce, Geraldine was approximately 3 years old when her parents married.

Geraldine's father, now in his late sixties, worked as an independent waiter in a rather sporadic manner, earned minimal wages, and was constantly heavily in debt. His history of chronic alcoholism and severe pathology (on occasion involving hallucinations and paranoid ideations) interfered with his functioning as a father, as a husband, and as a contributing member of society.

Geraldine's mother died of cancer at the age of 48, one week before Geraldine's eighth birthday. Verified history revealed the mother's pregnancy with Geraldine as very difficult because of the presence of many uterine tumors. She was hospitalized six days prior to Geraldine's birth, which was by Caesarian section. She also had a hysterectomy at that time, with a history of multiple fibroid tumors for several years. The mother had excision of papilloma, left breast, when Geraldine was about 4-1/2. Cancer was first diagnosed when Geraldine was almost 7 years of age, and the mother had a mastectomy of the right breast, at which time there was a marked involvement of axillary glands. She was again hospitalized for X-ray therapy, was home briefly, then was hospitalized for a left breast mastectomy. She had a rapidly metastasizing type of growth, with weight loss (her top weight had been 275 pounds), anorexia, vomiting, weakness, shortness of breath, and severe chest pain. She went to the Emergency Ward four months after her last surgery, was admitted, and died one day later.

The mother was described as having been extremely bright, a "whiz" at math, and employed in the accounting departments of several government offices. In personality, she was portrayed as a difficult, demanding, domineering, and stubborn woman. She was volatile and at times had an uncontrollable temper.

Early history was almost totally lacking because of the father's hazy and unreliable memory. Geraldine's mother stayed at home to care for Geraldine and tried to alleviate dire financial problems by caring for other babies and by sewing. She returned to full-time employment when Geraldine entered nursery school. The parents had violent fights, with many separations. The fights also involved Geraldine's half-brother, who left when she was quite young, and her half-sister who remained in the home. The wild fights were always very upsetting to Geraldine who was described as having clapped her hands over her ears and having run out of the house.

Following her mother's death, Geraldine stayed with her half-sister for one week, went to an aunt's for another week, and then moved to the home of a neighbor who had often cared for her when the mother was either working or ill. She remained at the neighbor's for a little over a year. The following summer she spent with maternal relatives on a farm and then, at the age of 9-1/2, went to live with her maternal aunt and uncle. She remained there until her treatment began, which was when she was placed at the Children's Aid Society, a residential treatment center for emotionally disturbed children. Residential placement during her analysis was considered essential to insure continuation of her treatment by offering her controls and stability which her relatives could not provide because, against Geraldine's wishes, her father would occasionally take her for visits with him. Neither Geraldine nor the father described what occurred on the visits, but they became increasingly upsetting to Geraldine and she eventually asked her aunt not to allow the father to take her away from the aunt's home. She also needed protection in the event that there was further exacerbation of the amnesia.

The causative factors in the onset of the amnesia are still only partially understood. The initial knowledge was that the amnesia had followed her deceptively having changed D grades in music to B's (she was an excellent student); that she had responded to a reprimand for the deception by running away for several hours; that she had received threats by her father of being sent away to a "bad girls' " school; that she had gone to school the following day and had failed to return home at the close of school that day. Only during the subsequent years were other factors learned which doubtlessly related to the grossly overdetermined causes of the amnesia. These precipitants included a weakening of her denial of sexuality and of her femininity upon seeing a school film on menses (she had forged her aunt's signature on the permission slip, too guilty to mention it); and a pelvic examination subsequent to the trouble at school because she had described a man following her on that runaway day. Other important events, revealed much later in her treatment, included her aunt's angina attack; her father's proposal that the two of them move to another state; his telling her at that time of her illegitimate birth; and a false report of the sudden death of her father which had been given to her by one of the father's friends.

When Geraldine had been found wandering in a dazed state, she had known neither who she was nor where she lived. She had said that she had a severe headache; she had realized that she was on the wrong bus; she had known that her mother was not with her; and she had asked a strange man to take her to a hospital. She had been returned to her aunt with the aid of the police. The father had had Geraldine hospitalized for complete neurological studies, and no organic basis has been found. She had then been referred to a child psychiatry clinic. At the onset of the amnesia, Geraldine had recognized only her father, then later her half-sister. She had had no memory of her mother's terminal illness and death. The eleven-month delay until her placement at the Children's Aid Society and the beginning of treatment had been due to the fact that no analytic opening was yet available.

The aunt gave a full description of Geraldine as she had known her. She referred to her as strong-willed and determined, with "lots of grit." She felt the closeness in their relationship had developed after the onset of the amnesia when she had remained out of school for the semester. Prior to the amnesia, Geraldine had been withdrawn and distant. She had never cried and had controlled her anger, although she had expressed it in looks of cold fury and in devious ways. She was of very superior intelligence and had artistic and musical talent (her mother had played the piano and had sung well, often participating in church services). Geraldine had been transferred to Major Work classes (for children of superior intelligence) when she was 10-1/2. Her amnesia had not affected her reading, but she had forgotten all of her math except simple addition. Geraldine had no close friends and chose only children whom she could dominate and rule. She was competitive and jealous. After the amnesia, she withdrew from peers completely.

REVIEW OF THE TREATMENT

Geraldine at 11 was of average height and of slightly stocky build, with beginning breast development and mild acne. Her complexion was light brown; her large eyes were intense and in no way shadowed her dark-rimmed glasses. Her shoulder-length hair was worn in two braids. She had an air of quaintness about her—in her dress but even more in her overall appearance. In conversation, she spoke voluminously with a vocabulary far advanced for her age, avoiding slang and with stress on propriety and impressing others. She often used literary references quite aptly and as proof of how well read she was. She presented herself as calm, self-assured, and in command of the situation. Her posture had a stiffness and rigidity. Most striking was her lack of true affect, and her deceptiveness at times through her effort to portray the affect which she felt was appropriate and expected of her.

Geraldine approached me and treatment with wariness, caution, and a manifest attitude of cooperation: she came promptly and talked incessantly. She set out to impress and to please me. Early in her treatment, she offered factual statements about her amnesia, describing its onset or saying, "I know my mother is dead, but I cannot remember it." Such statements disappeared as she tried to keep the amnesia hidden from all others: it was a defect, to be hidden and ashamed of. The most notable aspect in those early months was Geraldine's lack of any genuine affects, the frozen quality of her personality and the shallowness of her relationships.

The character of her relationship with me initially was clearly a need for my presence, which was most evident in her reaction to my three absences during that first year. While I was there, all was fine; when I was away, everything seemed very different and her self-control seemed to vanish to an alarming degree. Her need for my presence was gradually understood as her need to have me there to support her "proper girl" self. The origin of this was her tendency to adopt the behavior which various parent substitutes had expected of her and which, to a great extent, coincided with the ideal of a good daughter which her mother had held up for her (although she had failed to serve her as a model).

My first absence resulted in Geraldine's acting out an identification with her mother in her verbal attack on her father for his neglect, thus displacing her anger toward me to him. This outburst stunned the father. Geraldine had never spoken to him like that and "it was just as if his wife had returned from the grave." A few months later, I was away for one week and she repressed the approaching separation. But while I was gone, she was depressed, cried frequently, and had serious fights with the other girls in the cottage. Although these reactions frightened her, the most terrifying aspect was the extent of the emotional impact of my absence. When I returned, all was fine; she described affectlessly what had occurred and added reproachfully, "I don't understand it at all, and I don't know why I'm so certain, but I'm positive that none of this would have happened if you had been here."

I agreed that such strength of feelings did not make much sense unless we understood that they were not just of the here and now but were feeling memories from older times in her life. She had felt then that things got out of control when that very important person—her Mama—was not with her. Although she scoffed at such an explanation, there ensued the first meaningful discussion of her mother, a partial lifting of her amnesia. She told of the week following her mother's death when her sister had carried out the plans for Geraldine's eighth birthday party, plans that had been initiated by her mother. She said, "I know my sister Joanne was trying to cheer me up, make me happy"; and we could now talk of this reversal of affect, the "happy good mood" which was the affective counterpart of denial, a defense which, as I have already mentioned, was often employed by Geraldine. Her further talk of her mother was bland and affectless as she described how unavailable her mother always had been: "She did little for me as she was always either working or ill." However, in her poems and plays Geraldine presented repeated themes of loneliness and having to fend for herself. When we could view the clear loyalty conflict in one of her plays, true affect began to enter the sessions.

The fourth anniversary of her mother's death was now near and Geraldine told of her envy of her mother who had gotten chocolates Geraldine longed for but never could get and who could play the piano beautifully by ear while Geraldine had to learn to read notes laboriously. She had been unable to compete with her mother and had demonstrated this by dropping piano lessons. She became openly depressed and self-injury was evident in a fall and a painfully injured knee on the actual anniversary date of the mother's death.

As my summer vacation approached, Geraldine could never remember it, the dates or details, but negated my reference to her tendency to forget unpleasant things. This repression was accompanied by an intensification of all of her other defenses: denial, isolation, denial of affect, and rationalization. During my vacation, she became very upset, feared she would "crack up," and accused a male staff member of trying to kiss her. She wrote me an unmailed letter of reproach. Geraldine was experiencing added internal pressure at this time in that her menses had started shortly before I left for vacation. She could not even mention this to me and when I brought it up, her reply, "It's a perfectly normal, natural thing that happens to every girl sometime between the ages of 12 and 21," was bereft of any feeling. I asked if she had read this in a book somewhere and her shy reply was, "Sure, that's how I have learned most things." We could then speak of her turning to books, rather than to people, for answers and we could also identify this as her "learning through her head and not through her heart" (with feelings via a human relationship).

When I returned from vacation, she told me of the events which had transpired, but she had no feeling whatsoever. We could then see how, during my absence, she had become terribly anxious and out of control. When I came back, the crisis was over, she had lived through it, and the anxiety was gone. This pattern she repeated many times. And thus she often repeated her tremendous anxiety of being overwhelmed, of being annihilated, engendered by a fear that her needs would go unfulfilled.

A new quality of a positive mother-child relationship emerged in the treatment as she read fairy tales and sang lullabies to me. When I said that her Mama must have done such things with her, she disagreed with annoyance: her mother had been too busy.

President Kennedy's assassination brought forth her initial denial and incredulity of death news, then an appropriate but most intellectual description of her reaction. Her only affective response was to seeing the casket lowered into the ground. When I spoke of an earlier funeral—her Mama's—she vehemently denied that this was relevant. "I was too young, I knew nothing of Mama's funeral, I wasn't even there." The following week, she fell in the gym and broke her left leg, requiring a toe-to-thigh cast for ten weeks.

However, she missed only one treatment session, the day of the fracture. She described her trip to the emergency ward, her pains and fears. She expressed an unrecognized loneliness as she described the miserable day. Very soon afterward, she began asking me personal questions: where did I live, what was my home like? She reminisced about how her mother used to take her up "that hill" to the suburb where I live. She recalled how it used to seem to her "like going into a different world."

At Christmas, Geraldine spoke of having, for the first time in her life, a feeling of Christmas—of love—inside herself. Within a few days, she openly professed her deep love for me but could not bring into the analysis her subsequent frustration and anger engendered by my lack of reciprocation. It was at this point that a cottage parent's mother died of cancer and Geraldine was hospitalized overnight for severe abdominal pains, with no positive physical findings. She told me of her desolate loneliness in the hospital, negating that her longing was for me, and proceeding to displace her feelings for me to the resident at the hospital. She developed an open crush on him, wrote him notes, and at times chastized him for his double talk to her. My attempts to bring this into the treatment were met with vehement disagreement, criticism of me and the conclusion that I was "a nut."

Through the month of January she showed no anxiety about leaving elementary school. However, she fell twice the first week of February, her first week in the overwhelming junior high school. That was also the week in which her cast was removed. I reminded her of this pattern of not permitting anxiety ahead of time, her fear of being overwhelmed, having to get through the crisis and then letting her feelings out in some way. I went on to say that it must have been this way at the time of her mother's death, when she had had real needs and no idea of how they would be met. She furiously disagreed on the basis that her loss was minor since her mother had never been able to do that much for her anyway. (This feeling was omnipresent in the transference.) However, that night she sobbed unconsolably for hours, slipped and twice fell in the hall.

Geraldine was steadily becoming more upset; her old defenses were no longer effective. She regressed (was infantile in her play), isolated herself to her room, and withdrew from peers; her school work deteriorated; she was furtive and suspicious, and talked of seeing a man in a brown suit lurking around. I knew all of these things about her but not from her; with me she was angry, short, and sarcastic, refusing to discuss anything. She had a wild, out-of-control episode one stormy night when she crawled out the music room window, ran around the campus, and crawled into the senior boys' cottage, where she was found sleeping on the floor. Her diary explanation, which she sent to my office, was that she thought she was going crazy, that an adolescent boy, Carl, had made her go out, that she felt as if she were standing aside watching herself, and later realized that Carl was really part of herself.

I can only speculate on precipitates for this acting out of Geraldine's bisexual conflict, and the data for my speculations came only years later. A few days preceding this episode, she had seen a sex-education film at school, and the science teacher had asked for a volunteer in an experiment. Geraldine had volunteered and was to lift something from a can. The object proved to be the heart of a cow. She had been filled with horror, repulsion, and had felt ill. It seems clear that Geraldine denied affects and facts regarding sexuality just as she did regarding illness, surgery, and death. To her, growing up and becoming a woman meant being attacked sexually, being attacked surgically and dying.

It was quite soon after this incident, on the fifth anniversary of her mother's death, that Geraldine truanted, spent the day in a church, and reported taking forty aspirins over a three-day period. She would not discuss any of this with me (the aspirin taking, the trip to the emergency ward, the day spent in church, the truancy, and so on) but soon began to treat me openly like a mother, asking me what her dress size was and instructing her father to leave her birthday gifts with me. Within a few days, she had reversed her positive feelings for me to hate and had then projected them onto the other girls—they hated her, were out to hurt her, to kill her.

This behavior reached a height one day when she refused to leave school to return to the residential treatment center: she was not safe, was subject to attack, was mistreated, and she feared her amnesia would return. She was brought home from school by a cottage parent and came to her session looking horrible: drawn, tense, masklike. Walking in like a robot, she said, "I have taken all I can. I can stand no more." When I replied that this must be exactly as she had felt much earlier in her life, she began sobbing, "Yes, but it's five years now since Mama died. I should be over it, but I'm not. I want more than anything for someone to hold me tight and really mean it." She told, in detail and with tremendous affect, of her mother's final trip to the hospital, of having been told by Joanne of Mama's death. Joanne had told her that Mama had gone to join Jesus and that Geraldine would join her there one day. Geraldine had sat staring and Joanne has asked if she had heard and Geraldine had replied, "Yes, Mama is dead." She had not cried until that night at a neighbor's home; she had been afraid to cry lest she might not be able to stop. She recalled having cried for twelve hours, alone, without comfort or support.

Geraldine told of the funeral, the hymns sung, the trip to the cemetery, the adults discussing whether she should go to the graveside, and their decision that she was too young. Thus she had sat alone in the car. She explained she had not seen Mama lowered into the ground; the first time she had seen that was with President Kennedy. We talked of her longing for reunion with Mama (a merged relationship), of her taking the aspirin as a gesture which reflected this longing; yet this was not what Mama would have wanted for her. She was now 13, her needs for Mama were less than at age 8, she had capabilities, could do more for herself. After this, she was better able to deal with her positive feelings toward me—once offering herself to me in her wish to be my cat, to be loyal and loved.

A new resistance now emerged in the treatment: Geraldine refused to take in my words and was repulsed by anything I said. On the one hand, she showed an oral inhibition by missing meals, and, on the other hand, an out-of-control orality by eating paper in the sessions. I spoke of her inability to eat what she should, yet her reaction to my words was as if she were saying, "Don't feed me that line." She responded by narrating an early experience when she had foolishly made a hot dog, and, using her finger and a piece of paper, she bit herself. She looked repulsed as she added, "How can cannibals do it—eat humans?" I equated her affect with her response to my words, as if taking them in were devouring me as well, being cannibalistic. It was following this work that Geraldine for the first time seemed truly allied with me in the treatment. She progressed in many ways: showed increased self-esteem, evidenced a Negro identity which she had consistently denied, looked and dressed more like an adolescent, and was, in general, more attractive. Her domination of peers shifted to more genuine leadership, with an exchange of affection in her relationships.

Geraldine now also manifested a difference in her reaction to my summer vacation. She showed no repression. She was angry with me and equated my trip with her mother's "trips" to the hospital. Her mother, she said, had always deceived her. She had never spoken of cancer, had told her she was going to the hospital for an examination, yet had always returned having had surgery. Geraldine voiced these complaints with annoyance and irritation, a preamble to a later expression of stronger aggression toward her mother. Yet these complaints were memorable as the first nuances of direct angry feelings toward her mother. Her own guilt and defense of undoing were discernible as she told how her father had drunk and worried her mother, as if worry caused cancer. In contrast, she had avoided worrying her mother by helping at home and by getting very good grades.

There was also a gradual change in Geraldine's relationship with her father. She became openly glad to see him and was eager to meet some of his relatives who were visiting from a nearby state. She made her father a birthday card, then quickly and guiltily made one for me. Thus there appeared, in the transference, the first oedipal jealousy with concomitant guilt and the need to atone. Geraldine's guilt still prevented her from identifying with her mother, but she began to identify with her aunt by an interest in cooking and by working with younger children at church.

Geraldine's progress was interrupted by the very serious and for some time undiagnosed illness of her aunt, the one who was so meaningful for her and with whom she had lived. She repeated her earlier denial of illness by asking friends into the home on one of her regular Sunday visits and thus acting as if her aunt were feeling fine. I pointed out this repetition to her and she acknowledged that she was terrified; her aunt "looked like a ghost." She had thought, "Here it is again. Where will I go, where will they send me?" She felt like running away, but where? This acknowledgment led to her recall of events preceding the amnesia: her conviction that her aunt would die when she had had an angina attack; her memory of her father's proposal to take her away to live with him in another state, and his disclosure then of the fact that the parents had not married until she was 3 years old. She described how she had suddenly felt that she did not care about anything and as though her head were held on by strings. It was after this partial lifting of the repression that, for the first time, Geraldine recalled the woman with whom she had lived during the year following her mother's death. Her conclusion about this return to the repressed was "I am getting help."

Her aunt's physical condition improved, but she then had a relapse at the end of December and told Geraldine she expected to enter the hospital for tests during that week. That same day she also reprimanded Geraldine for secretly wearing lipstick at church and expressed strong disapproval of Geraldine's forwardness at church with an adolescent boy with whom she was infatuated. Simultaneously, Geraldine experienced two other very upsetting events. She visited her father's apartment for the first time in two years and saw evidence of the fact that his lady friend had recently moved in with him. This was a repetition of earlier experiences of having been rebuffed by her father. Now he had a lady friend living with him and Geraldine was again "out."

Earlier, the father had seductively encouraged her ideas of living with him and keeping house for him after her mother's death but in reality had clearly offered nothing. Then again, prior to the onset of the amnesia, he had proposed that the two of them move together to another state. It seems clear that Geraldine's oedipal guilt was intensified at the time of her father's rebuffs. In the treatment, she was extremely upset by my news that I would be leaving the residential treatment center, even though she knew intellectually that her treatment would not be interrupted. Again, she could voice no anxiety about any of these events, yet acted out the anxiety by running away, taking Sominex, and appearing late that night at the hospital emergency ward, asking for a reevaluation. She told of her worry about her aunt's health, her fear of cancer, and her feeling that her birth had been responsible for her mother's illness and eventual death.

Subsequently, Geraldine refused to talk with or visit her aunt, declaring that her aunt's heart could stand no more, that she had already caused her aunt enough trouble. I interpreted her identification with her aunt, explaining that she had heard of her expectation that she would go into the hospital and that she had then brought about her own trip to the hospital, as if what happened to her aunt also happened to her. Now in the sessions, Geraldine excluded me and tried to hurt my feelings—employing again her defense of reversing passive to active. She feared she would contract epilepsy, saying good people did not get epilepsy, and equated illness with loss of control to a murderous degree. In her sessions she acted like Jesse James, but refuted her own murderous thoughts and subsequent guilt in relation to me. While negating all interpretations, she tentatively acknowledged the existence of the unconscious (referred to by her as "things in the back part of my mind") in her discussion of her slips of the tongue, described by her as "skid talk"—a topic which was being currently discussed in her English class.

As Geraldine again became friendlier toward me, both positive and negative oedipal elements appeared in the transference. She was jealous of me in reference to her father: he always seemed so eager to see me, so hurried to end their visits so that he could spend time with me. Then she displaced her excitement with me onto the girls at school and described how embarrassed she had been when they had hugged and kissed her after her original song had been played in a school program. She said she wished that she could avoid the girls and "all that excitement." When she missed her next session with me, I pointed out her displacement and her concomitant avoidance of excitement with me. To this she replied, "You're a nut—a real nut."

Geraldine reacted strongly to the fact that she was the only Children's Aid Society child whom I would continue to see after my job change. She was excited and elated at being my "chosen child" yet filled with guilt. We could relate her concept of "chosen child" to its popular equivalent in that an adopted child is often referred to as a "chosen child." This stirred her guilt about eliminating her competitors, that is, the other children, and also stirred her loyalty conflict. Her wish to be my chosen child meant being disloyal to her mother, to her aunt, and ultimately to her own race. In her fantasy, it also represented being male in that she thought she would literally come with me and that I would be working with boys in the adolescent residence which was housed in the same building where I would have my office. She felt she would live there and would have to cut her hair and wear boys' clothing to be acceptable to me.

With the approach of the sixth anniversary of her mother's death, I mentioned Geraldine's failure to say anything about this. Her angry retort was: "What do you expect me to do, celebrate?" But once more she brought nursing books and renewed her interest in becoming a nurse, this always having occurred as an undoing when her aggression toward her mother became strengthened. Her father then requested a birthday visit to his home and, on the day following his request, Geraldine fainted in school. She confirmed my suggestion of a connection between these two occurrences by telling of many early trips with her father to various churches, where wild orgies took place and "women were fainting all over the place." That was a time when she was terrified of her father but this no longer was true. She wanted a visit but felt that attending church with him was not a good idea. The visit went well.

With me, Geraldine became increasingly disappointed and frustrated by my not doing enough for her. These feelings were now displaced onto her young, male French teacher. In one session, she performed for me the interpretive dance that she had choreographed to the song "Somewhere." She took the part of "Len," treating me as her partner, and the dance represented a search for love, love of a mother. The next day in school she had a panic reaction, fell, backed into a corner, and felt as if she were being stabbed. I interpreted her reaching toward me in the dance as reaching toward a mother, as well as her disappointment, deep frustration, and killing (stabbing) wishes. Her guilt ultimately resulted in her feeling that it was she who was being stabbed. This led to her musing about the incident a few months previously, when she had taken the Sominex and had gone to the hospital. She said she was "truly glad" that had happened because it had brought about a change in her: prior to that she had felt like "half a person" and that whatever happened to someone dear to her was happening to her. Suddenly she had realized that she was Geraldine, a separate person, and that the Sominex would have hurt her.

Subsequent analytic unfolding included many references to the superiority of males. Geraldine wrote a poem as if depicting herself as a tall, lanky farm lad; she identified herself with the soldiers in Vietnam. Her original songs were songs of love —search, unworthiness, declaration, rebuff, reunion—in which a strong male identity was apparent. And we could now discuss her belief that being male meant being first and crowding out all competitors, including her father, for her mother.

Geraldine's anger about being female was basically directed toward her mother but appeared in relation to her sister. Joanne's advanced pregnancy was the impetus for revealing her fantasies in respect to conception. She said she knew that the father determined the sex of the baby. She knew that with her brain. Yet she still harked back to her earlier belief that the mother had the baby and controlled the baby's body formation: sex, coloring, and so on. We could then look at her conviction that it was her mother who denied her the "number one status," that is, to be male. She often referred to herself through her parody of a national car rental advertisement: "I'm number two, but I try harder."

Geraldine's anger at her mother as the source of her femininity emerged in the transference several months later. We were discussing Joanne's uterine hemorrhaging, or, more accurately, I was verbalizing this, while Geraldine sat in icy silence which reflected her controlled rage. She then reproached me for giving her "nothing good, only the bad." She wanted nothing from me: no news, no explanations. "Female troubles" were repulsive to her and she wanted to know nothing of Joanne's physical condition. At the end of this session, as she scooped up her books and papers, she took my ballpoint pen. She was embarrassed the next day when I inquired about this and apologized for forgetting to bring the pen back. She continued to forget it, finally lost it, and later replaced it with a pen she had begged from her father. We could see her strong need for something from me, who gave her nothing. And I suggested that she had earlier felt this way about her mother.

Geraldine's aggression to women increased in many directions. She was angry with her aunt for not extending an immediate invitation to her upon the resumption of her (Geraldine's) relationship with her. She was hurt and furious because Joanne did not tell her directly of her son's birth. She was jealous of her 18-year-old girl cousin when the latter visited her aunt for the summer and used her old room. She became angry at her father's lady friend when she saw the robe this woman had given him for his birthday; such an intimate gift seemed to shatter her denial that their relationship was a platonic one. She proceeded with her requests for visits with her father and her aunt two weeks before my vacation. She was angry with me about the vacation and wished "much wrath on my head."

Geraldine had these two visits and became very upset. She saw her nephew for the first time and was most offended because her sister had subtly prevented her from holding him. The next day she swallowed three safety pins (my unspoken thoughts were of diaper pins), one of which had to be removed surgically from her esophagus. When she returned to treatment, after her two days in the hospital, I interpreted to her her aggression toward the introject. I spoke of how earlier it had seemed that when something happened to someone else, it seemed to be happening to her. This seemed to be the other side of the coin. Her anger toward others was taken out on herself, as if it were not happening to her at all but to someone else instead.

Geraldine was definite about not wanting any visits while I was away. She felt discouraged about her treatment but was buoyed up by my speaking of how she had gotten through difficult times before and could again. The last day before my vacation, she brought her guitar, sang the Beatles' song "Help," and smiled when I said I felt I had gotten the message. She added, "Sometimes I can sing what I cannot say." She managed well as a model citizen while I was away.

I have given some fairly detailed accounts of the first two and three-quarters years of Geraldine's analysis to illustrate the quality of her object relationship and how its development via the transference made mourning possible. The ensuing three and three-quarters years followed more typical analytic unfolding. She engaged in relatively little acting out, showed increasing tolerance for anxiety and an ego capacity to involve and ally herself in the treatment. She now became my sole source of information; and she brought material, albeit at times with much resistance. External reality events (illness of her sister and of her father) ushered in regressions for brief periods, but these regressions never reached the point of a merging with the object.

Sequentially, the analysis unfolded with many ups and downs. There was a period of resistance, this time anal in form. For a time, Joanne then became a focus for her ambivalence. As her aggression toward women became more conscious and more tolerable, she had less need to deny it in action, that is, in being good instead of bad. Originally, this need to be good had taken the form of being a very good student so as not to worry her mother. During this period of our work on her aggression toward her mother, her grades declined markedly. Later they rose but this time not as a defensive maneuver.

After more work on her bisexual conflict and on her oedipal rivalry, Geraldine no longer denied her sexuality. She began asking for sexual information, stating that for one who was sixteen, she was grossly naive. She produced many of her sexual fantasies, the majority of which emerged more readily after I had given her a bit of factual information.

Primal scene material entered the treatment via dreams, screen memories and, later, through transference manifestations. Only after this work was Geraldine truly able to learn the details of her mother's illness. She had condensed the two mastectomies into one, yet was puzzled because her recollection involved two separate apartments at the time of surgery. She asked for clarification by way of doctor's reports and hospital records. This clarification of the reality was indeed helpful to her as she was then able to recall more details of the timing of surgery and the places where they had lived. Thus memory of the two separate mastectomies returned.

Typically adolescent, she worked at arriving at her standards and choices regarding many things, including the choice of a church; which was preceded by a period in which she was an agnostic. As for the type of racial identity which was "right" for her, she "knew she was no Uncle Tom," and finally concluded that she was aggressive for blacks' rights but not revolutionary.

During the process of adolescent object removal (A. Katan, 1937) as she moved into dating, she spoke of the conflicting standards in her background. Her mother had married twice, had lived with her father, had had her, then had married him only much later. Her identification with this aspect of her mother became apparent in her strong identification with a friend who thought she was pregnant. Geraldine told of having morning nausea, adding, "Who ever heard of a pregnant virgin?" and it was she, Geraldine, who fainted when the friend found that she was not pregnant. When Geraldine had first heard of the friend's suspicions of being pregnant, she had been shocked, had disapproved, and had spent several days crying uncontrollably in her sessions.

She could see that her degree of affective reaction was out of proportion to the current reality and agreed to a connection with her first knowledge of her mother having been unmarried when she had become pregnant and of her illegitimate birth. Her tears could then be understood as a piece of her mourning—her mourning the death of her idealized mother when she had learned from her father the circumstance of her conception and birth. This information had followed the actual death of the mother by two and one-half years and had preceded the onset of her amnesia. We could also gain some insight into a major determinant in her symptom of falling as an identification with the "fallen woman," her mother.

Geraldine also talked of her father's double standard: he lectured her to be a "good girl" yet he still failed to marry the woman he had been living with for years, "just like with Mama." Her aunt represented severe morality: she was extremely rigid and considered card playing, dancing, dating before age 18 as all evil. Geraldine decided, "I have to look at these standards of others and come up with my own."

Her reactions to separation and loss occurred several times with favorite teachers as well as with those staff members of the residential treatment center when she moved, at age 16-1/2, to a group home for twelve adolescent girls. Of course, the end of her analysis loomed steadily during the final fifteen months of treatment, even though she predicted that she would be in touch with me in the future (which she has been). She was able to deal with these losses with most appropriate affects. When the termination date was about four months away, she had three brief periods of amnesia (called "lapses" by her), two of them occurring as she left my office. In our discussion of these "lapses," we could see how the old pain of loss (the fear that the feeling was too great) was intolerable since she not only felt nothing, but she knew nothing—the blank of amnesia. These three incidents took place within a two-week period and did not reoccur.

I might conclude with some of Geraldine's reflective comments during the final months of her analysis. As to her many struggles with her aggressive feelings and how she dealt with them: "With Mama, I was scared to death to step out of line. I saw with my own eyes how she attacked, in words and actions, my Dad and sister and after all I was just a little kid—very powerless." And, "Mama didn't treat Dad too well at times. I remember once when I was about 5, he was hospitalized with pneumonia. We moved and Mama didn't even tell him because she was mad at him." Another description of her dilemma was: "How could I ever be mad at Mama; she was really the only security I had. You really have to side with the parent who looks after you."

Geraldine had always known that her mother was regarded as the black sheep by all of her relatives and that she, Geraldine, was never thought of as a person, only as "Helen's daughter." In her early years, relatives were never around or interested in her, and her aunt had taken her in, after her year with the family friend, more from a sense of family duty than because of any genuine love for her. She recalled that her aunt could never tolerate "back talk" and she was convinced that her aunt could know if she had even an angry thought. But Geraldine was equally in touch with the positive factors in these relationships. She spoke of her gratitude to her mother for imbuing her with a love for music, and reading, both of which were great pleasures in her life. She was realistic about her aunt, "We will always disagree on many things; my aunt is old and won't change and, after all, she has a right to her own opinions too." Her aunt's husband she had always regarded with fondness and admiration; she admired his sensitivity, patience, and industriousness.

As to her earlier denial of all affect, again Geraldine's own statements are more descriptive than any I might make. "You know, I think my treatment, or really my life, has been sort of in three phases. At first, I blotted out all feelings—things happened that were more than I could endure—I had to keep going. If I had really let things hit me, I wouldn't be here. I'd be dead or in a mental hospital. I let myself feel nothing and my thoughts were all involved with fantasies, fairy tales, science fiction. Then, in the second phase, my feelings took over and ruled me. I did things that were way out. And in the third phase, now, my feelings are here, I feel them and I have control over them. One of my big assets is that I can experience things, with genuine feelings. At times it hurts, but the advantages, the happiness, far outweigh the pain."

Her reflection on her relationship with me she expressed when she brought her boy friend to meet me, several months after ending her analysis. She explained that she had told her husband-to-be all about herself, her life, her treatment. She referred to me as her friend, then turning to her boy friend, she said, "She never lectured me, blamed me, chastized me, praised me—she let me be me, she helped me to know and to sort of like myself."

Her gains were notable in this period of adolescence, when she had to try to accomplish the developmental tasks as well as the major task of mourning a loss which had had to be blotted temporarily from her memory and which took along with it the capacity to feel herself worthy of living. Life events will help determine her future since her tendencies toward somatization and action under great anxiety remain, although they are under relatively good control. Many aspects of this lengthy analysis I have, of course, excluded in my attempts to focus on the task of mourning which was accomplished via the transference.

BIBLIOGRAPHY

Freud, A. 1960. Discussion of Dr. John Bowlby's "Grief and mourning in infancy and early childhood." *Psychoanalytic Study of the Child* 15:53-63.

Freud, S. 1917. Mourning and melancholia. *Standard edition*, vol. 14. London: Hogarth Press, 1955.

Furman, Robert. 1964. Death and the young child: Some preliminary considerations. *Psychoanalytic Study of the Child* 19:321-34.

Katan, A. 1937. The role of "displacement" in agoraphobia. *International Journal of Psycho-Analysis* 32:41-50.

Evolution of the Transference in the Psychoanalysis of an Adolescent Boy

Carl P. Adatto, M.D.   *New Orleans*

In this presentation I shall attempt to demonstrate the evolution of the transference, and its correlation with the infantile neurosis, in a boy with petit mal epilepsy who began his analysis with me at age 14 years, 10 months, and terminated eighteen months later.

The analysis of the transference of the adolescent occupies the same central position as it does in the adult patient in psychoanalysis, and is subject to the same standard analytic technique. With the adolescent, one must reckon with how transference reflects his level of development and the radical restructuring of his psychic apparatus. The formerly stabilized psychic structures and well-defended intrapsychic conflicts become instinctualized, with regressive changes in function en route to a more general resynthesis of the psychic apparatus of the adult. Concurrently there is a reduction in the availability of those autonomous ego functions which are basic to the capacity to be psychoanalyzed—especially the functions of self-observation, frustration tolerance, reality testing, and the ability to free associate. With diminished capacity to free associate, there is a reduction in the amount of data that lends itself to effective interpretation. Loewenstein's (1972) recent clarification of the role of the autonomous ego in analytic technique is applicable to the adolescent. A task of the analyst is to assay and utilize the autonomous functions in the therapeutic alliance, and to keep within "tactful" limits as he gathers and interprets the analytic material. The capacity of the patient to recognize and utilize transference in interpretations depends on his capacity for self-observation.

A specific aspect of the psychic transformation—the change in the nature of object representations—is clinically observable in the data of this case. The impact of castration anxiety, and change in the body ego which comes with the resexualization of the internalized parents of the superego, is a phenomenon of crucial importance, and is often underestimated in the analysis of adolescents. Hypercathexis of the genitalia and body creates a state in which there is a relative withdrawal into the self and a simultaneous lessening of transference interest. The ebb and flow of the castration anxiety often is paralleled by the state of the transference or the degree of narcissism during the course of the analysis.

Recently I postulated (Adatto, 1971) that the capacity for effecting a *transference neurosis* is less well developed in the adolescent than in the adult (and better developed than in the child) because the capacity for displacement, primarily and centrally, from the internalized parental object to that of the analyst depends on the full maturation of the psychic apparatus. As a consequence, the transference neurosis, which is so useful in the analysis of an adult neurotic patient, is less completely available and more tenuous in the adolescent. Geleerd (1957) stated: "It is self evident that the adolescent does not develop a transference neurosis like the adult patient" (p. 268). She also noted that the handling of the transference reactions, which coexist with the relationship to the analyst as a need-satisfying object, is different from that of the adult capacities and the more the real parents as need-satisfying objects are used as resistance. I believe that, by patiently and carefully timing the interpretations of the transference, these obstacles can be overcome sufficiently to conduct a productive analysis.

Freud (1912) stated: "The part transference plays in the treatment can only be explained if we enter into its relations with resistance" (p. 104). His later elaboration of the theory of aggression and its relationship to negative transference (1937), together with his explanation of resistance in structural terms, broadened the theoretical underpinnings of the concept of transference. For instance, the need to analyze the negative transference in the adolescent becomes even more imperative if one understands its significance in relation to the unbinding of aggression which accompanies the transformation of the superego, as well as to the decathexis of defenses. Also, transference can be conceptualized as being utilized as an ego defense within the analytic setting. This factor calls for its interpretation as a defense as well as for the analysis of its genetic connections. The necessity for distinguishing the negative transference from a narcissistic retreat into the self offers a further challenge to the analyst. In the adolescent, negative transference and narcissism often appear indistinguishable from one another until the patient's associations belatedly clarify this difference. Inaccessibility of the obscure negative transference can easily lead to a therapeutic impasse, a point considered in this case. The analyst, by viewing the adolescent in terms of his maturational tasks and capacities, can be better prepared to decipher the transference presented by the patient and make effective use of it in understanding the nature of the neurosis as revealed in the transference, and in the analysis of the neurosis through transference interpretations.

In my opinion, parameters (Eissler, 1953) to standard technique at times are indicated in adolescents as they are in adults. Parameters are last-resort measures when free association and interpretation have been exhausted. However, care must be exercised lest the introduction of a parameter lead to an impasse or a premature termination of the analysis. In this case, there was occasion to contact the parents at certain points of the analysis, which coincided with resistance to the analysis by the patient (and also obstruction by the parents, on which I cannot elaborate). The fact that the patient was suffering from epilepsy and needed medication, and that his mother and father were divorced, created a difficult family situation which readily lent itself to resistance. Prior to the termination of the analysis, the oedipal threats the patient felt from the mother, and the lack of "protection" from the stepfather, paved the way for a major resistance which proved to be unanalyzable. At that point, I decided that it was preferable to adhere to the use of interpretation and not become involved with the parents, even though interpretation turned out to be insufficient to keep the analysis going. My feeling was that any deviation from analytic technique would not be interpretable later, and thereby would harm the boy's opportunity for further analysis at a later date.

THE PATIENT'S HISTORY

The patient, Jack, originally was referred for analysis at age 12 because, since the onset of epilepsy at age 11, his schoolwork had deteriorated and he had been presenting some behavior difficulties at home. He had had a two-year period of analysis which had been interrupted when his analyst, a woman, moved to another city. At that point, I saw the patient for further analysis.

Jack had a sister two years older, and, when he was 4, his parents were divorced. His mother moved with her children to a city distant from the father, and she reported that Jack was subsequently depressed, that he cried and hugged his pillow, apparently in response to the separation from his father. However, he remained in contact with his father, spent long periods of time with him each summer, and the father continued to take an active interest in his son. The father remarried and had children by his second wife. The mother remarried at about the time the patient's first seizure occurred at age 11. Another problem in his infantile period was the fact that Jack soiled until age 6, a problem for which the parents sought guidance. On one occasion, he had become extremely upset when he was administered an enema, following a period of constipation. Apparently there had been no serious observable problem until the onset of his epilepsy. He had been found crawling about the floor, confused and unable to recognize anyone. He could only remember doing his homework and, the next thing, being in bed. The neurological examination was within normal limits. An electroencephalogram revealed features consistent with both grand mal and petit mal epilepsy, and nine additional tracings during a five-year period showed no significant change. He received many types of anticonvulsants, but was lax about taking them. Most of his ictal episodes were petit mal in character, although there was a history of some nocturnal generalized seizures.

Following the seizure, Jack's behavior became difficult to manage at times. He would provoke his sister, mother, and stepfather into anger. At times he would goad his stepfather into spanking him, and capitalize on his subsequent guilt. When physical punishment was abandoned, he continued to make his anger known by yelling and banging doors, then would feel remorseful and make amends. His academic work was creditable until this period; it then became characterized by spotty performance to the point of near failure.

I shall not discuss Jack's first analysis other than to note that he worked through sadomasochistic aspects of his neurosis, that there was an effective construction of his enema trauma, and that later he was able to bring his masturbatory fantasies into the transference, with resultant satisfactory analytic work. The beneficial therapeutic effect experienced during this period of analysis paved the way for motivation for his analysis with me. While he was in better touch with his inner life and neurotic difficulties, he nonetheless had the task of engaging in a new transference relationship.

THE PSYCHOANALYSIS

In his first session with me, Jack came to my office exactly on time but he felt that he was late. He was burdened down with

school books and seemed to be in a pleasant mood. I was immediately impressed by his clean-cut, almost pretty features and
the overt passivity with which he presented himself. He complained of having to take Industrial Arts instead of Mechanical
Drawing because there were not enough students enrolled in the
latter course. This meant that he had to take Industrial Arts a
second time and he stated that he was rather poor with his hands,
especially in planing wood. Evidently he did not get along well
with his teacher because he was clumsy in handling tools. Aside
from not having been assigned to the French teacher whom he
preferred, he stated that the rest of his courses seemed to be
satisfactory. He announced, after these preliminaries, that he now
had a girl friend whom he had met during the last several weeks of
his summer vacation. He had been corresponding with her since
coming home and felt very pleased with this relationship. I
gathered from what he told me that this was one of the reasons he
was in such a good mood. From his description, he seemed to have
the adolescent love feelings usual in such a situation. He told me
something about his relationship with his father during this past
summer. His father had not bothered him too much except on one
occasion: when his cousin Amy had visited, his father had insisted
that he take Amy to a party instead of Mary, his girl friend. He
complied because he had to take Amy whether he liked it or not.
He went on to describe that he was unhappy about his former
analyst having left him in the "middle of things," and told me that
he had expressed his displeasure about this to her. Then he wondered about how often I would like to see him, explaining that he
would like to turn out for football this fall, and he asked if I could
arrange his schedule in such a way that he could do both. Obviously it was impossible to do both; he seemed to be quite aware of
this and to be challenging me to see how I would handle his
request. He presented the problem in coming to analysis, or
resuming it with me, as one of being forced into a position without
having much say about the matter. This he stated so categorically

that I pointed out to him that if I encouraged him to play football, I would be ignoring his problems; and if I insisted that he come in for analysis, I would be in the position of telling him what to do. I suggested that it possibly would be best if we postponed the discussion of the frequency of his visits until the next session, as our time was up.

There were two major themes outlined in this session which became evident during the first two months of analysis: the preoccupation with the loss of his first analyst and a readiness to enter into a struggle with me as he had done with his father in respect to being told what to do. Rather than dealing directly with the theme of the lost analyst, he went into detail about his summer girl friend, Mary, their correspondence, and the lack of this. Even later in the analysis, I was not able to do much by way of connecting the loss of these two people because he himself insisted on keeping them separated. In regard to his father telling him what to do—forcing him—he related a seizure he had had during the summer in reaction to an incident in which he expected his father to get angry with him for arguing with his stepmother. He was pleasantly surprised when his father was not angry, but instead had considered the situation to be humorous.

Jack agreed, in his second session, to enter analysis with me. About a week later, he informed me that he was going away on a scout officer training expedition over the weekend. He evidently liked scouting and had been a member of a troop which had received commendation for the speed in which it put up a camp site. He told me that troop discipline was getting stricter, and that he would have difficulty in going to parties on Friday night because that was the night on which the troop met. Because of the meeting time some of the boys had dropped out. In a joking way, he said that they had a new scout master who was more lenient than the older, rigid one. They frequently enjoyed breaking the rules—going off for hamburgers when they should be putting up the tent or building campfires—and in general making life miserable for the younger scouts. It was with considerable glee that he told me of the hazing that the younger members would get on camping trips. He then went off into some thoughts about tying people to trees or putting them in pits, or about the ways in which they set up traps to catch pigs in the fields. A considerable amount of affective reaction accompanied his tales and he encouraged me to participate in finding out more of the details of these activities. He described his membership in the Sea Scouts as something rather bland in contrast to the regular scouts, and he told me that they had had their Sea Scout activities on a boat which had been sunk and now was salvaged and worked over by the scout troop. He made a disparaging remark about the man who originally had owned the boat prior to the time it was sunk.

A more direct confrontation occurred the following week. When Jack arrived in the office, he immediately notified me that he had not as yet received the snapshot of Mary; however, he had received letters from her and was happy about that. Next he announced with pleasure, that he had got a 95 in a Civics paper which he had written and which dealt with his German ancestry. Previously, he had told me of having got a 90 in another French examination, but later had told me that this had been the lowest grade in the class. This time, he said, there were no "buts." Then he asked me if I had been the one to request an electroencephalogram on him. Apparently this was a way of finding out how active a part I planned to take in matters pertaining to his epilepsy. Actually, he knew that I had made no such request. He then reported that he had discussed scuba diving with the neurologist and had received permission from him to dive. After some long silences and lapses, I asked Jack if he had been dreaming, for he seemed to be in a reverie. He asked me which I was interested in, day or night dreams, and that all he had were day dreams about being with Mary. It seemed that he had some reluctance to talk about himself, which I pointed out to him. He was rather surprised that I was aware of this, and went on to discuss, with some concern, the mother of one of his good friends, who was depressed. Upon leaving the office, he checked with me again about changes in the schedule which we had made and expressed pleasure in the fact that he would have an easy time getting to his sessions.

Another kind of mood in Jack's sessions was playfulness. He came into my office one day with some false teeth, made of paraffin gum, in his mouth. He told many jokes, as before, and gave some addenda to the elephant series of jokes with which he was occupied. As he was chewing his teeth, he expressed thoughts of "chewing out" people, and he associated better than he had ever-done previously. He talked about cannibalism, people eating each other, cutting each other up, what a big joke it might be to eat someone. He told me of a teacher who called him to task in class when he was drumming on his desk and mimicked the teacher's anger and exasperation, recounting how he naively played dumb, saying words to the effect, "Who me?" Evidently this was a technique which he used freely with adults, and he let me in on the actual workings of it. While the joking mood prevailed, I pointed out to him how it appeared that he had been doing the same sort of thing with me. He cocked his head to one side and, with a smile, said that he saw no evidence for that, adding that he was not worried about my "shoving" him out, something which he had expressed at another time. He recalled that, for as long as he could remember, he had had the tendency to provoke his parents; then he would become fearful of reprisals and of being ejected from their presence.

During the early part of his second month of analysis, Jack had sessions on two successive days which produced associations about masturbatory activity among his scout friends, and the initial signs of his coming close to experiencing intense anxiety in my presence. This led to his first reported dream in the analysis, which heralded his moving toward the transference as a resistance, and to a long-standing fear of bodily mutilation.

Upon entering my office, he reported that he planned to go on a scout trip that weekend, and again he went through in detail the initiation rites of tying boys down, pretending to shove them off the cliff, and the like. When he had been initiated, he had been blindfolded and given a club with which to hit another one of the boys; and he had ended up in some sort of mock battle. Once during an outing, one of the leaders had pretended to be bitten by a rabid dog. There had been much commotion and all of the scouts had been frightened until the joke was revealed to them. However, he, Jack, had begun to catch on that it was a joke shortly before they told the truth by reason of the fact that the allegedly bitten person had not been rushed to the hospital and the leaders had waited first to eat their ice cream. Repeatedly Jack conveyed the idea that he mistrusted adults.

When he alluded to sexual activity in camp, he commented that he never had seen any masturbation openly performed; he did not demonstrate much anxiety in talking about his own masturbatory activity. He mentioned how one boy, prior to the time he had gone camping, had been threatened with having his pubic hair shaved off with a straight razor, but that this procedure had since been outlawed. Previously, he told me that one of the older boys had asked a younger one for some Vaseline and had to tell the younger boy "what the score was" in regard to masturbatory experience. He did not have much inclination to discuss homosexual activity. Further association led to his telling me how one of his stepfather's friends had needed a tracheotomy recently because of a chest collapse. He also told me of two hernia operations which he himself had had as an infant. He had no memory of the surgical procedure other than what he had been told about it, and he described the large scar he now had on his abdomen. During this past summer he had felt a strain and pain in the scar and had been worried lest he have a recurrence of his hernia. At this time, he reported that recently he had noticed that one of his testicles was lower than the other, and he asked me what that meant. Then he told of the money that he received for his sixteenth birthday, but that he also wished he had received some gifts as well as money.

Jack was considerably subdued following his previous session, commenting that he had a cold, and then reporting the first dream which he had brought into his sessions with me:

> I was in a German concentration camp as a prisoner in a cell. The guard was watching me but got out of sight so I climbed up to a window and escaped out of it. Two other guards came looking for me. One went one way, but I met the other one coming around the corner. He had a rifle and shot me, grazing me on my behind. Then I took a broken bottle and attacked him, jabbing him in the throat and face and cut him up until I killed him.

Jack had few spontaneous associations to this dream except for the fact that he wondered who the German might be. The recall of an association he had had concerning a school theme which he had written about his own Germanic origin, brought him to thoughts of his father. As he talked about his awareness of his thoughts about men in general, and his father in particular, such thoughts involving attack and physical damage, his anxiety became manifest. However, he collected himself and commented that he hoped it did not rain over the weekend during his outing.

The following session, Jack associated to acting as the middle man in a love affair between two of his friends, a boy and a girl. "Girls can be awfully pushy with boys—but not when it comes to being sexy." As he talked further, he added that girls could be aggressive sexually as well. After a pause, he said, "Someone who saw me coming here thought I was your son," and laughed at the mistaken identity. Then he asked me what my middle name was and how to pronounce it.

Jack failed to arrive for his next appointment. This marked the start of a pattern of approaching affectively charged associations, as a result of analytic work, and then moving into the transference as a resistance—in this instance as a resistance to analyzing his homosexual sadomasochistic conflict. When a transference failed to serve the resistance, as evidenced by overt anxiety, he would miss one or more sessions. He would resume his analytic work when his associations and actions were interpreted.

Another important development took place in the analysis shortly thereafter. Jack had a petit mal seizure while talking to me. Five other times, during the analysis, he lost consciousness in my presence, and, in addition, he reported an episode which had occurred in school. These six instances were the only ictal episodes which he reported during the course of the analytic work, and apparently he had no other episodes in or out of the analysis. From the viewpoint of the transference, it seemed that these episodes were a means of handling intense anxiety in relation to me, which developed during the course of a session and could not be contained at the time. I considered this to be a way of removing himself from me much in the same way as he did when he would not appear for his sessions. The epileptic symptoms, appearing almost exclusively in the analytic situation, could be explained as a manifestation of transference neurosis, and also as a temporary massive regression of ego functioning in the face of overwhelming anxiety.

The first of the petit mal episodes took place at the end of Jack's second month in analysis. When he came to the office, he was pleased to report that he had finally heard from Mary who was sorry that she had not written him earlier. We discussed more about dating and this led to his revealing his actual interest in looking at girls and their bodies. There ensued a flood of recollections and reporting of events that had happened in his life over a period of time. At age 5, a cleaning woman's daughter had exposed her genitalia to him. He added that *she* was almost caught by her mother in the act. Several years previously, two girls and one of his boy friends had gone to one of the girls' houses where the girls had exposed themselves to the boys. He stated that he would not expose himself in either of these instances. This led to information about his having peeped at his sister's genitalia on many occasions; the last period of these frequent episodes had taken place during the previous summer when he could view her through a crack in his bedroom wall. While he was relating this material, and apparently groping for a word to describe the crack in the wall, he reported that he had just experienced a seizure. Apparently he had been out of contact for five or ten seconds, but there had been no evidence of convulsions. Following this seizure, he seemed detached for some time, and I commented on his detachment and how the seizure, or "spell" as he called it, might have been a way of handling his intense feelings about what he had just revealed to me. He reacted to my intervention by becoming again alert.

Following this session, Jack's associations were banal, and, for some time they dealt with the trivia of his everyday life. I confronted him with this observation whereupon he asked me if I believed that he was withholding information. I told him I had no direct evidence of that, but that it was likely he was concerned with matters in addition to those about which he was reporting. Associations led to apprehension about his sexual interest in girls and his involvement, for a brief period, in forming a "fraternity" of boys which was designed to cope with girls. Next, he talked about two current girl friends, Cindy and Ann. He apparently was engaged in erotic play with both of them, and after describing some details of this play to me, he missed two appointments without notifying me.

When I met Jack in the waiting room at his next appointment, he was looking around at the walls in a comical way, feigning that this was the first time he had seen my office. Upon coming into the office proper, he wore a foolish grin on his face and said, "Well, why don't you ask me?" He launched into an elaborate explanation of how Thursday's football game had been delayed because a player had broken his wrist and of how he had had to wait for the ambulance. As a result, he had been late in coming to my office, and by the time he was two blocks away, he had realized that there were only ten minutes left. And so, he had not come at all.

The following day as he was leaving for my office, Cindy stopped him to tell him something important about their relationship. "She told me that I was lying on top of Ann at a party," but he said this was not quite true. In a dramatic way, he showed me how he had been sitting in a chair with a pillow in his lap and how Ann had been lying on the pillow in his lap. Then he told how he had got caught in a dark room with one of Cindy's girl friends. The girl's father evidently had turned the light on unexpectedly, while he and the girl had been kissing and hugging. He seemed rather pleased with himself as he talked about this, and made a mocking gesture of throwing his arms up in front of his head as if to ward off imaginary blows from me. Then he told me of an argument with Ann in which she had accused him of treating her as though she were a toy which he took out of its box, played around with a bit and threw away, only to pick up another toy. At the time he had taken her keys away from her and when he had not immediately returned them, she had threatened to go home and sleep with him since she could not get into her own house. This was followed by more risqué jokes which he delivered entirely in a one-sided way. He had become totally immersed in himself.

The following session Jack reported a dream: "It was Mardi Gras and many boys and girls and I were all dressed in night gowns and house coats. They were all dressed in similar clothes. Jane was also there." He said that Jane was Cindy's cousin and he wondered about being dressed like a girl, alluding to his recent thoughts about what it would be like to be a girl. I suggested he might feel that if he got too involved with Cindy he would turn into a girl. Immediately he responded: "Yeah, if I get too deep." Then he laughed at his double meaning. He missed the following appointment and stated that he had been home playing football with Jane. He, Jane, and another boy had beaten five other boys in the game. This was typical of the way in which Jack would bring in productive analytic material, miss appointments, and then subsequently introduce new information. Next he revealed his intense sexual interest in girls and their anatomy. For instance, he told me that a girl friend had told him that she had had a dream in which he had a baby who was calling him poppa. He asked me if she might have meant that he was going to give birth to a baby and was rather confused in his fantasies about birth and the question of whether he was a mother or a father. However, he decided that since the baby had called him poppa, he was probably the father in the girl's dream.

It was also now evident that Jack was bringing his analysis into his everyday life. Concurrent with this were his reports of blowups at home, his growing defiance of his parents and his teasing of his sister to the point where fights broke out between them. He told me that as a joke he had thrown a small book at his mother, that it had accidently hit her on the head, and that she had got so angry she would not give the book back to him. At this point he had begun to struggle with her physically, whereupon his stepfather had broken up the wrestling match. When the incident had cooled off a bit, he had thrown the book at his stepfather, with the result that he was punished by confinement to his room. On several occasions during the analysis, I received calls from the parents regarding similar behavior and, in a general way, I informed them that we were working on the meanings of this. They seemed more or less content with the fact that Jack was trying to understand his behavior. These parental interventions seemed not to bother Jack overtly, but we soon came to see that he was trying to draw his parents into the analysis as another means of avoiding the analytic work. He knew that if he became belligerent at home, his parents would get upset and possibly call me.

After approximately four months of analysis, I confronted Jack with his pattern of missed appointments and with the fact that I was having a hard time understanding him. He retorted by saying that frankly he felt he was coming to the analysis only because he had been forced to do so from the beginning. He stated that he had been taken to his first analyst by his mother directly for the appointments and he did not have much choice; but now that no one checked on him, he was handling it in his own way. The following session, he reported a dream: "I was going to a dance and as I was going in, Bill Stark was coming out." He associated this dream to the actual events that had taken place during the dance, and to meeting a new girl. Evidently Bill had come to pick him up and bring him home as he was walking out. He was enamored of his new girl friend, but also reported his interest in Bill and some other boys. There was some hint at this time of his awareness of some homosexual feelings which were of a kind different from the Boy Scout type.

This foregoing session was followed by four straight absences. I called Jack's home to contact him, but his mother came to the phone and told me that he did not want to come to his sessions. She believed the reason was related to some disagreements over financial matters which she had been having with Jack's father. However, Jack later called me and said he had been busy and would be in for the next session. He arrived on time and was in a friendly mood. We discussed his absences and failure to contact me, and the effect on him of my having talked to his mother. He explained that he was trying to work out some problems at home by himself but would not go into these to any great extent. Again he stated that he felt he was being coerced into the analysis and that he would prefer to solve his problems on his own. At this point, I had the impression that he was actively testing me. I told him that I respected his right to analyze or not, and I requested that he, himself, let me know if he were not able to come for his sessions. I notified him that I would take absence and silence about it as a sign of his wish to discontinue the analysis. He then added that one of the causes for his unhappiness about coming was the fact that he was discouraged because he could not drive an automobile because of his epilepsy. (The state law permitted driving at age 15.) He wanted to know if the analysis would help him in overcoming his epilepsy, and he wanted some assurance from me on this point. From the way in which he presented this to me, it seemed that he wanted to bargain with me about the analysis. After a lively exploration of his thoughts about the analysis, he indicated that I understood him when I told him I thought that the real current problem in the analysis might be that he was afraid of some build-up of feelings toward me. After that, he rarely missed an appointment, but he was frequently late—a pattern which had not been marked before.

A few weeks later, another productive session took place: Jack started by wondering whom he should take out to a dance. The theme of tremendous uncertainty as to with whom he could pet, and which girls he liked, was investigated. Then he compared me with Cindy as someone he really liked and in some ways felt sure of, yet he was afraid to get too involved with her because she was willing to accept him as a person. He went on to tell me about a party to which he had gone over the weekend, and of the fun he had had with several friends. He and a girl had thrown peanuts at each other. A peanut had hit his eye and had burned him for a while. He then looked at me rather seriously and stated, "I know you are going to say that the peanut means something else and that you will pick up on that again." He said that before he had begun missing the sessions, he had become irritated at me for trying to get at some of the underlying meanings of his actions. This had bothered him a lot. We discussed why this might have bothered him, how it was similar to behavior he attributed to his father, and how "getting into" his inner life had been rather threatening to him. He accepted my explanation and commented that what he had talked about was not in the same class as "just analyzing a thrown peanut."

The analysis became more intensive from this point on, and sporadically Jack was able to bring together his current life situation, dreams, and transference which centered around his sadomasochistic conflicts. Displacements from me to other people occurred. He came to one session with a small, neighbor boy friend, who remained in the waiting room. Upon entering the office, Jack showed me his report card and discussed his poor school performance. I commented that both his bringing the friend to the session and discussing his schoolwork seemed to me to be leading him away from more important considerations, and I wondered if he felt the need for some distance. He made several sly remarks indicating partial acceptance of this, and immediately discussed his relationship to his (male) French teacher for whom he evidently had strong positive feelings. He told me that this teacher had called him and asked if he needed any help, to which he had replied in the negative, explaining that the good grade proved that he needed no help. His next associations were two dreams:

> I was walking by school. Two of my classmates were running out as though they robbed the place. The police came up and grabbed both of them. One policeman branded each boy with a hot iron. It made a hole in his forearm and it became swollen and red.

His first association was that these boys were considered "hoods" and were not really as tough as they think.

> I was riding in a car with my father. I drove it up to a hospital, got out, and the gang of boys beat my father up and carried him into the hospital dead. During the fight, I also got out of the car. I was knocked down by a boy when I tried to help.

He said that he had been getting along well with his stepfather, that he certainly did not want to kill him, and that his real father recently had been hospitalized with an illness. In reflecting on his own associations, he revealed a long-standing fantasy that the engorgement of his erect penis signified that it was injured.

The following day Jack had a petit mal seizure while reciting his lesson to the French teacher. Several weeks later, he reported that when he had gone to a music concert with his teacher, he had left during the intermission to be with a new girl friend. Then he told me about girls who wanted to touch boys' penises. He indicated awareness of the underlying homosexual implications in his relationship with the teacher and of the connection of the teacher with me. Subsequently, he became aware of the pervasiveness of his sexual feelings toward everyone he knew and of his intense interest in his own body.

In a later session, I indicated how much of his earlier material had shown some feeling that I might harm him if I knew how he felt toward me and others. I noticed that, while I was saying this to him, he became sleepy and rubbed his eyes. At this point, I commented that his sleepiness might indicate that he wanted to get away from me. He took sharp issue over this with me, saying that I was not correct and that he did not feel that I was a menace to him. He reported that his previous analyst had made the same mistake in making incorrect assumptions about him. I stressed my lack of knowledge about him and how, of necessity, I had to make many guesses and ultimately depend on him to find out how he really felt. Toward the end of the session, he told me that he had been actually experimenting with me, as he had done with his first analyst on former occasions, by trying to get me to ask him many questions. He commented that as long as I would be active in asking him questions, he could more easily talk about his feelings toward me; if I waited for him to do this on his own, he found it practically impossible to initiate the discussion of his feelings with me. During this exchange, his sleep state had changed to one of alertness; he subsequently became more frank and assertive toward me.

In the next session, Jack expressed concern about his father's health, and associated to my going away for a few days, and his anger at his first analyst for taking "monthly trips." He began to talk more about his relationship with his father, how he looked forward to being with him in the summer, and yet how much he also hated this. He associated next to guns, talking about the fun of shooting a shotgun in the summer and the fact that he had no gun of his own. With a grin, he looked at his genital area and said, "That is, I don't have a shotgun." He told me of a friend who was an excellent shot and used a gun well. He paused a second and then reported that he had had "a spell." This permitted us to connect his feelings to his father and to me with his feeling about his own genitalia. He responded by talking about having gone with a friend on a hiking trip on which they had met some girls and had engaged in some petting.

As we entered further into his conflict over his passive wishes for me and his fear of genital damage, the transference intensified and the associations to earlier periods of his life increased. Four concurrent sessions will serve to demonstrate this.

Jack opened the first of these sessions by saying that he had thought he would be late and was surprised that he was on time, since he had been talking to Cindy about some of their negotiations regarding sexuality. He had a syringe in his hand and kept playing with this during the session. Then he began talking about taking dope and, at one time, made a gesture with the syringe to symbolize a penis sticking out of his pants, threatening me with it. He said that he was looking forward to a party on Saturday night and hoped that Cindy would be coming with him as his date. He definitely planned to "make out." He joked a great deal about sex and engaged in a bit of talk about some of his previous sexual episodes and of his earlier sexual experiences. He told me that he found he was no longer afraid of his stepfather and realized he had not feared him for some time. Evidently, he had been having a struggle with his mother in regard to cleaning up his room. He reported that she had walked into his room that morning and said to him, "You had better be the housekeeper of this room." He had replied, "O.K.," and had continued with what he was doing, commenting to me that she must be out of her mind to think he would clean his room. He presented a dream: "I was going downtown with John to get a fishing reel and was also supposed to go some other place and was not sure that John would go with me." He associated to this dream by saying that actually he and John were going to get some fishing reels and that was why he had cancelled his appointment with me one day before he had taken his hike. This led to the problem of his reactions to me and his avoidance of me. At this point he grinned and said he had something in his blood—morphine. Again he played with the syringe, and once more talked about this being a gun and his penis. In an even more mocking way, he raised the syringe from the vicinity of his groin, put it into his mouth, and squirted it. At this point, he laughed rather heartily, spit out, and began putting the syringe in and out of his mouth as though to mimic eating. He was playful and relaxed.

The main theme in Jack's next session consisted of his pleasurable anticipation of the party and his hopes that Cindy would come to it. He talked rather extensively about his genitals, his sexual behavior, his fantasies about petting with Cindy; and at this time, he spoke openly about fellatio—his wish that Cindy would suck his penis. He was referring to the previous session and seemed to be demonstrating a continuity between sessions more markedly than he ever before had done.

In the following hour, he noted that Saturday night had been a flop. Cindy had not shown up; she was supposed to have come with Fred, who was the president of the club. Jack had tried to kiss another girl but she had slapped him. Then he told me some joke about what was "his clawed hand like," the answer being that his clawed hand was like an eagle, only five times as strong as a "bird," referring to an outstretched middle finger. Jack manifested a jovial mood despite his weekend disappointment. He spontaneously volunteered that he had had no dreams. As he left he said that he remembered he had left his constitution at school, explaining that this was the United States Constitution. He laughed, realizing the double meaning of the word and said that indeed he did have his constitution, pointing to his groin.

In the fourth session (of this series) I discussed with him a visit which I had had with his parents and which had been prompted by their concern about his defiance toward them. Jack seemed to be happy about the outcome of the visit. Then he told me a joke about masturbation. Had I heard about the canoeist who had taken two strokes and had shot across the lake? He proceeded to talk about his masturbatory fantasies in a way much freer than previously, and reviewed his masturbatory history, from his earliest memories at about 4 or 5 years through his more recent episodes in which his sister, Mary, Cindy, and others were fantasy objects. He told me about a time, while he had been in analysis with his former analyst, when he had had a masturbatory fantasy regarding her and had felt uneasy and anxious about this. It was clear to me, at this point, that he was building up considerable anxiety and that the anxiety in respect to revealing his masturbatory activities was far more threatening even than that attendant on the revealing of his fellatio fantasy. I told him that I felt that he was quite anxious at this time and that he had had spells in my office previously under such conditions. He continued by talking and joking about his sexual thoughts of Cindy, and in a short while he reported that he had had a partial seizure. The episode lasted a short while; he was not totally unconscious. It was both surprising and pleasing to him to have discovered that he had retained consciousness. Following this, he demonstrated a slight amount of confusion. His next association was that he was going to see his French teacher and talk to him about some of his studies. There was further discussion of masturbation at this time and he told how he had a homosexual episode some years previously: three boys had got together, undressed, and one had "shoved his penis up" the other boy. Jack himself had tried to shove his penis up one of the boys but had failed to get an erection. He had had mutual masturbation with one of these boys when they spent the night together and often they had talked, during their masturbatory play, about sexual activity with girls. He spoke again of his relationship with his sister when he had been between 10 and 11 years of age; on occasion they would get into bed so that he could masturbate her. She, in turn, would merely look at his genitals and not masturbate him. He said that the last time he had seen her genitals had been at their summer home; he could not peek at her any more since the walls and doors were now tightly closed.

Following these sessions, Jack showed much interest in his anatomy and physiology in reference to scuba diving, and he asked me for general information particularly in regard to pulmonary functioning. He reported his generalized feeling of well-being, his erotic activity with two different girls, and his general curiosity about his own and other people's bodies and functioning. Two events—an accident he had witnessed, and my impending departure for two weeks—elicited the following data on two successive days. This was as closely as he ventured to analyze his positive oedipal wishes.

Jack was about twenty minutes late. He had thought that his bike was in the garage at home but had realized that he had left it at Tom's house, so he had taken a streetcar to my office. He reported a dream which he declared to be unusual:

> I was playing tubular bells in a band, hitting them out of tune. Also I pulled a string in the middle of a number which made a ringing noise like a telephone. Everyone, including the band director, was surprised. The band was below the stage and on the stage the principal of the school was presenting an award to an old lady. I went up on the stage and poked her with my hand. When I realized what I was doing, I pretended to faint and fell to the floor.

Associations came with difficulty. The old lady was like his mother, only, he stated, he was not even angry with his mother. The bells made him think of the wedding march. The manner in which he described the poke at the lady was like the joke which he had told me about the clawlike hand and the extended fingers of the "bird." He said that he had masturbated the other night but was reluctant to discuss his fantasies other than by saying that he had visualized having intercourse with Cindy. He commented that from the dream he sounded "like he is out of tune" with someone. Then he proceeded soberly to tell me about an incident which had occurred while he had been playing baseball the day before. One of his friends, Jimmy, as a result of a collision had sustained multiple injuries—fractured ribs, a punctured lung, and a ruptured spleen—and had almost died while in the operating room. At the point at which he was trying to recall Jimmy's hospital room number, he experienced a petit mal seizure which lasted momentarily. When he recovered from the seizure, he engaged in serious analysis of the antecedent associations, connecting these with his apprehension during my presence. As he left, he shrugged his shoulders and wondered what he would dream of next.

Jack was late for the next session. He brought with him a book on scuba diving and went into detail about the laws of physics which apply to diving. Toward the end of the session, he got up and asked me to look at the back of his shirt to see if it was wrinkled, for he was perspiring rather profusely. He followed with the comment that he was rather tired and proceeded to lie on the couch; he seemed happy, although uneasy, and began to whistle a tune. Upon leaving he commented that he would like to use the couch again when I had returned from my trip.

From this point on, he used the couch more or less regularly, more often than not sitting up, turning around with his feet toward me; he expressed the feeling that by using the couch he was being more adult. On one occasion, he told me that he had a girl friend who went to a psychiatrist and he (the psychiatrist) had told her to lie on the couch. He commented: "She said she was not going to get laid by any psychiatrist,'' whereupon he said that this girl had come to me at one time but subsequently had gone to the other psychiatrist because I had no time in which to see her. He told how he had been trying to pet with Cindy but was getting nowhere. He reported a dream: ''There was a girl in school who had her hair dyed blond and under pressure brought it back to normal color. In the dream she was blond again.'' He described this girl as promiscuous and then told a story of a 9-year-old girl who had been seduced by a 25-year-old man. At this point, he began to light matches rather vigorously, and associated to his French teacher who had asked him to help decorate his apartment, which request Jack had refused. He reported that he was continuing to tease his mother, simultaneously seeming to be attempting to tease me with tales about his French teacher. He told of his masturbatory thoughts about Cindy and other girls as well as open erotic play with them.

Subsequently, Jack developed interest in the mental workings of his friends and other people, obtained a summer job in a hospital, and began to interrelate with his peers in a more playful manner. Some of this behavior appeared to be an exhibitionistic means of allaying his sexual anxiety: he would incur resentment and arouse the girls' curiosity by telling them risqué stories or by performing such actions as, for example, pulling a condom out of his pocket before them. One day, while sitting in the chair, he said he was afraid of falling asleep. He reported a weekend of intense orgy-like activity with a gang of girls and boys at a resort; they had jumped into swimming pools with their clothes on, had aroused the police, had masturbated, and had awakened people in the middle of the night. It seemed that at this time he was not only experimenting with his feelings but also becoming freer in testing his feelings with me. In contrast to his former attitude, he seemed to care little about my opinions; now he asked for none of my opinions and, rather flamboyantly, was displaying his sexual prowess.

There was further intensification of Jack's transference as he moved deeper into his sadomasochistic fantasies and the connections with earlier periods in his life, especially his identification with his father from whom he was separated. He could feel little protection from his stepfather in regard to his assertive aims toward his mother, and to some extent his sister. This made it increasingly difficult for him to live at home, and he spent a great deal of time with his friends. He indicated that he wanted me, through intervention, to "protect" him from his mother, and from his oedipal strivings toward her. He was able to get in touch with his passive wishes toward his father when he was unable to contain these in the transference and had taken a trip with a 26-year-old male friend of the family. The eroticized aspects of his relationship to this man surfaced and frightened him. This experience permitted him to differentiate between the fantasies he had toward me and the potentially dangerous acting out with the young man. Following this episode, he was much freer in exploring his reactions to me as these related to his father. However, his angry feelings toward the mother were only superficially analyzable in the transference. Prior to visiting his father for the summer, he reported the following dream:

> I walked up the stairs in school without my shirt on. Then I went into my teacher's office, said "hello" very casually, and went on into school. I was hot and sweaty but felt very pleasant.

He was able to see the transference aspect of this dream in preparation for his visit with his father, but, more significantly he recognized that the "hot," "sweaty," and "pleasant" feelings originated within himself and were directed to several different people.

DISCUSSION

This patient was able to work effectively in his analysis as evidenced not only by his ability to subject his infantile neurosis to ego scrutiny and synthesis, but also as evidenced by structural changes: improved reality testing, increased accessibility to his drives, alterations in his superego functioning, and better frustration tolerance. His object relationships showed more age-appropriate characteristics, even though their infantile coloring remained.

At the beginning of the analysis, the patient had been engaged in resolving his transference to his first analyst, a woman. It was not possible for me clearly to understand how and to what extent this resolution took place, but there was strong evidence that it was associated with a separation from a summer romance with a girl of his own age. Comparisons between me and his first analyst occurred several times during the analysis, especially at that time in which the analysis of his resistance to the continuation of the treatment led to his revealing an experiment in provoking both me and his first analyst into answering his questions. While there were many determinants involved in this bit of analytic material, his change from sleepiness to alertness seemed to indicate an active mastery of his anxiety during the confrontation with me, and a step forward in the separation of himself from the objects represented by both of his analysts. It is noteworthy that in his first analysis, during early adolescence, his anal sadistic conflicts were more accessible than during his later analysis with me. The clear emergence of his mid-adolescent phase brought his genital conflicts to the surface, even though pregenital aspects were still evident.

The development of Jack's transference to me seemed to be accelerated subsequent to his exposure to his anxiety during the analysis of his recollection of having seen girls' genitalia. This led to an epileptic seizure in the office, one mode which he had of reacting to a dangerous situation. I feel that the transference to me, as the castrating father, served the purpose of resistance to the analysis of his own sadistic aims. As some of his sadistic conflicts were analyzed, he moved more toward the use of the transference as a central resistance to the analysis of his castration anxiety. Often he would display alternating shifts between the positive and negative aspects of his oedipal conflicts. For instance, he would turn his attention to girls and his mother when his relationship to males or the homosexual transference became threatening. Conversely, he would seek refuge with me or his male friends when he became too anxious with females. Thus, the transference was both a refuge and a threat as well as a way station in the process of the resolution of his oedipal conflict. At one point in the analysis, his fellatio fantasies indicated the emergence of oral conflicts which he apparently handled without much anxiety, even though his oral aims were in part directed toward me. The defensive aspects of these fantasies became clear when the subsequent analysis of masturbatory fantasies involving girls evoked sufficient anxiety in my presence to precipitate a seizure.

The confinement of Jack's seizures to his analytic sessions could be considered to be a form of transference neurosis, but also to be an extensive ego withdrawal in the face of overwhelming anxiety. The seizures were a complex psychic and somatic defensive activity. One cannot help but wonder about the history of traumatic events in his life, perhaps anteceding his enema trauma, because of the resemblance of the seizure episodes to a traumatic neurosis. However, the analysis yielded no information in support of this theory. Even though from time to time the transference became central in his life, he would obscure its intensity by displacement onto other people, by avoidance and by other defenses, and by that lack of sustained involvement in the analytic work which one sees in an adult patient who is immersed in a transference neurosis. Attenuation of the transference neurosis rendered the adequate analysis of the negative transference especially difficult. Missed sessions had multiple determinants; in particular: the avoidance of anxiety, narcissistic withdrawal—an interest in himself outside of the analysis—and the expression of negative transference. Upon resuming contact with me following such absences, he would evidence, through his associations, which determinant was in the foreground.

Toward the end of the analysis Jack recognized his homosexual feelings for me as transference. He could gain this recognition when these feelings were displaced onto a man ten years older than himself. The analysis of the displacement enabled him to distinguish between his transference aims toward me (and their genetic connection with his father) and the reality of the analysis. This resulted in further separation of the concept of himself from the concepts of me and his father. The functioning of his reality testing and observing ego prevailed at this point in the analysis.

The analysis terminated several months after the period reported because of Jack's lack of motivation to continue. This lack of motivation was clearly based on his reduction of anxiety, his decreasing tolerance for living with his mother, and his wish to reunite with his father. These manifestations, coupled with a clear-cut distancing from me, left the analysis with loose ends. I believe that the adolescent has a tendency to reintegrate his psychic apparatus more rapidly than does the adult in analysis, for the adolescent is in a more phase-specific state of rapid psychic progression. More and more, I am impressed with the adolescent's difficulty in dealing with the aggression that is unbound as the superego undergoes alterations, with the resultant intensity of a negative transference. Both the psychic reintegration and the presence of free aggression affect the evolution of the transference: the former by withdrawal of cathexis from the analyst, the latter by a more intense cathexis of him, which can be intolerably dangerous to the adolescent. While the transference was active, this patient engaged in sustained analytic work, and through the analysis of the transference he was able to analyze a segment of his infantile neurosis. In my experience, this sequence of intense and productive analytic work, followed by a marked diminution in the analyzability of the transference and by massive resistance to further analysis, while not necessarily the rule, is not unusual in the adolescent patient.

BIBLIOGRAPHY

Adatto, C.P. 1971. Developmental aspects of the transference neurosis. In *Currents in psychoanalysis*, ed. I. M. Marcus. New York: International Universities Press.

Eissler, K.R. 1953. The effect of the structure of the ego on psychoanalytic technique. *Journal of the American Psychoanalytic Association* 1:104-43.

Freud, S. 1912. The dynamics of transference. *Standard edition* 12:121-44. London: Hogarth Press, 1958.

——. 1937. Analysis terminable and interminable. *Standard edition* 23:216-53. London: Hogarth Press, 1964.

Geleerd, E.R. 1957. Some aspects of psychoanalytic technique in adolescents. *Psychoanalytic Study of the Child* 12:263-83.

Loewenstein, R.M. 1972. Ego autonomy and psychoanalytic technique. *Psychoanalytic Quarterly* 41:1-22.

The Analysis of Masturbatory Conflicts of an Adolescent Boy with a Note on "Actual Neurosis"

Jules Glenn, M.D.   *New York*

Masturbation conflicts are among the hallmarks of adolescence (A. Freud, 1958; Blos, 1962). With the increase in drives characteristic of this developmental phase, the teenager finds himself impelled to seek discharge of his sexual urges but fears the consequences of giving conscious recognition to his wishes and fantasies. Many adolescents succeed in resisting autoerotic behavior but fall victim instead to symptoms that result from failure to discharge. Tension builds and symptoms which have been called "actual neuroses" (Freud, 1894; Spiegel, 1958; Blos, 1962) may appear. Masturbation fantasies find expression in acting out (A. Freud, 1949) or in symptom formation (Reich, 1951; Freud, 1909; Arlow, 1953) which are compromises between the ego, id, and superego. In addition, portions of the desired masturbatory experiences, the act itself, or its fantasied physical consequences, achieve wishful expression in symptomatology.

The analyst will see before him a suffering individual such as the boy I shall describe in this paper. As I eventually learned in the

I wish to thank Drs. Mary O'Neil Hawkins, Isidor Bernstein, Milton E. Jucovy, Harold P. Blum, Maurice R. Friend, Herbert Urbach, Julian L. Stamm, Eugene H. Kaplan, Alan J. Eisnitz, and Melvin A. Scharfman for their valuable suggestions regarding the clinical and theoretical material in this paper. I also want to thank Mrs. Albert Sax for her editorial help.

course of his analysis, this boy's symptoms involved complicated compromises between his erotic and aggressive wishes (that ordinarily would have been partially dissipated through masturbation) and his superego's punitive demands, which were modified by the defensive activity of the ego. My patient's fear of being bitten by a horse had a structure similar to, but more complicated than, Little Hans's (Freud, 1909). His fear was an expression of his intense wish to bite sexually and aggressively as well as of his need to be punished for his illicit desires. The latter were displaced from primary familial objects and projected onto the horse. His fantasy that he would die following the bite resulted from a need to experience an orgasm and from the resultant diminution or loss of consciousness which he expected. He further anticipated death as a punishment for the forbidden climax. My patient's "hazy feelings" were also symptomatic, disguised expressions of sexual excitement, but they included defensive and regressive elements.

The analyst who recognizes the patient's struggle against masturbation and the resultant pathological formations must, of course, analyze the patient's fears, defenses, and wishes. If he succeeds, the diminution of symptoms may be marked, as in the case I shall present. He must also recognize the danger inherent in the possibility that the patient may well imagine the analyst is seducing him, urging him to masturbate. He must be careful not to be in fact seductive, in order to ensure that the patient's fantasy may at some point be analyzed.

I shall not present the entire analysis of this adolescent but rather shall confine myself to a period of several months during which the problems that I have outlined came into focus.

CLINICAL MATERIAL

Before describing the details of the analytic sessions in which this boy's masturbation was dealt with, I shall outline the pertinent factors in his disorder and the relevant analytic trends. From the outset, treatment comprised four sessions per week. In its earlier stages, the analysis was conducted within a face-to-face situation, that is, with the patient sitting up. During his fifteenth year, Billy assumed the supine position on the couch.

Following several years of analysis for a severe obsessional disorder, Billy at 16 was relatively asymptomatic. A tic, which had been prominent at the start of treatment, occasionally reappeared. He still tended to procrastinate and thus did not do as well in school as he might have. Since procrastination and withholding had now become characteristic features of his behavior within the analysis, we both suspected that he had progressed as far as he could at this time and that treatment might come to a close. The emphasis in this discussion was on the possible consequences of his procrastination; we did not plan a termination or interruption. However, as we will see, unconsciously, Billy took our discussion to mean that we would end treatment even though no date was set. At one point, Billy mentioned June as a possible time to terminate, but no date was set. We also discussed the fact that when Billy went to college in another year, treatment would inevitably end.

As June approached, Billy developed an intense fear that he had been or would be bitten by a horse, contract hepatitis, and die. The intensity of his panic was extreme, but despite this, he continued to engage in schoolwork and to maintain his usual good relations with his many friends. Although at times he thought that perhaps he actually had been bitten, in general he was aware that his fear was of a fantasied event. But that knowledge did not relieve his acute anxiety.

Before we came to realize that his obsessional fears were related to masturbation anxiety, Billy and I were able to analyze a number of its other determinants.

First, we learned that the appearance of these severe symptoms was clearly an unconscious attempt to prevent the termination of the analysis. Billy recalled that he had thought we might end treatment in June, but now, he said, that was "out of the question.'' He was so ill, he might even be unable to leave home and go to college. We were then able to understand his rage at separating from me, his feeling that I was leaving him and neglecting him as he had felt deserted by his parents in early childhood. After one such separation from his parents he had achieved toilet training. His struggle against soiling and other manifestations of rage were significant aspects of his personality and expressed themselves in his symptomatology. Obviously his procrastination and withholding were character traits which had resulted from his defenses against his anal sadistic strivings.

Billy and I also discussed his marked sexual attachment to me. The transference, now intensified by the threat of separation, had a strong sadistic component. This underwent repeated analysis throughout the treatment.

The fears of being bitten had begun shortly after Billy had played a practical joke at a girl friend's house. He had alarmed her parents by placing a toy facsimile of horse manure in the middle of their living room floor. Billy and his friends were delighted by the grownups' shock at discovering what they thought to be a serious mess. The following day, Billy saw a policeman on a horse and began to worry lest the horse had bitten him. This symptom spread to include other horses and grew in intensity.

It was not difficult for me to show Billy that his fantasy of being bitten, and hence killed, was an expression of his expectation that he should be punished for the sadistic act contained in the practical joke. He could see that his attack on the adults was a displaced attack on me, the deserter, and motivated by an anger which he feared to experience toward me directly.

We also spent considerable time discussing events in Billy's life which had resulted in his difficulty in evaluating what was real. As a precaution against further failure in reality testing, I suggested to Billy that he sit up rather than lie on the couch at this time, a suggestion which he accepted.

Despite his apparent excellent analytic insight, Billy's panic not only continued but even increased in intensity, with only brief periods of relief. It seemed likely that more analytic work was indicated; and, as we shall see, there were clearly additional, sexual factors associated with Billy's fear of horses and hepatitis. Since at this point we are reaching the crux of the masturbatory problem, I shall now proceed to describe individual analytic hours in some detail.

In one session, Billy described his resentment in response to his mother's failure to call the doctor when he had a sore throat and fever. She "stalled," did not believe he was ill, and let him suffer. But, he postulated, maybe he had brought on the fever to hurt himself. He suddenly became afraid that somehow he would be killed by formic acid, which he had used in school, or by urine which would enter his mouth as he showered. When he then said that I had told him such a disaster might occur, I explained that I had not said this, that, in fact, I had once told him he could not be harmed in such a way. Relieved, he informed me that his father had evaded his question as to whether he could be injured by urine.

I now reminded Billy that he had, in a recent session, mentioned a dream about a shower. Thereupon, he reported the dream more fully:

> I am taking a shower with a woman. I am afraid to touch her breasts. She would object. But she allows it. I am then watching television in a neighbor's, Mrs. Y's, room.

After describing the dream, Billy said that I, the analyst, would think that the woman in the dream was a neighbor. But, Billy said, she was not; she was really his mother and Mrs. Y was merely utilized to disguise this fact. Through this tortuous, obsessional reasoning, he was able to deny that it was either of these women. As he spoke of fantasies involving this dream-woman, Billy became increasingly terrified that he would die. He agreed with my interpretation that he had sexual desires toward Mrs. Y and that he feared death as a punishment for these wishes. He became calmer, and was able to describe daydreams in which Mrs. Y was a prostitute who bought condoms. Maybe he was interested in her body. Once he had spent the night at her house and had had trouble sleeping, fearing he would contract syphilis. After I had again pointed to his fear of punishment for such wishes, he recalled that, while lying on his parents' bed, he had feared that "something" would hurt him, something like a sexual attack. Toward the close of this session, I told Billy that teenagers may have desires to do something to a girl or woman and yet not know exactly what they want to do. Nevertheless, as did Billy, they feared punishment for these desires.

The next day Billy blamed both me and his mother for not taking proper care of him. Again he recalled that his mother had delayed taking him to the doctor for a sore throat and fever. Maybe, he repeatedly insisted, with mounting fear, maybe he would die of hepatitis. I explained that his fears derived from his guilty conscience and he retorted that I thought he was thinking about Mrs. Y. In fact, he admitted, he had been thinking of her—of her breasts and the shower dream. He also daydreamed that she was with a boy friend who then left her. She was a prostitute and he, Billy, touched her breasts. Then he paid her five dollars and they went to bed together.

After revealing this fantasy, Billy once more became terrified. This time he feared that his parents would kill him, or, that his brother would murder him because he had been jealous of him at his birth. His father had actually threatened to kill Billy when he had attempted to hurt this sibling.

Billy returned to his thoughts about Mrs. Y and another neighbor with whom he fantasized going to bed, but became upset by the possibility that not only his parents, but I, too, would hurt him.

In the following session, Billy again told of his fears of hepatitis, of constipation, and of being killed by me. As his thoughts turned to Mrs. Y, he said that he could see how, when he became angry or had sexual feelings, he would develop a fear of punishment. He recalled, with a great deal of affect, how an aunt with whom he had stayed when he was young, had threatened that God would punish him if he were bad or dirty. At the end of the session, he requested that we have an extra appointment on Sunday (something we never had) because he felt so nervous. When I did not comply, he became angry.

In the next session, on a Monday, Billy recalled his desire for the additional appointment, attacked me further, and feared that he would die. He announced that we could "forget about stopping the treatment for a long time" since his fears were so acute and irrational. This thought reassured him and he expected that his symptoms would now disappear. We both agreed that they served to forestall termination.

His fears, however, continued in their full intensity. He worried that contact with dirt would cause hepatitis. I reminded him of his aunt's threats that if he were dirty or bad, God would punish him. He must have thought, I suggested, that the punishment would be death. Billy replied that he felt his parents had reinforced these expectations. Repeatedly in this session he became angry at me for not paying full attention to him. His anger mounted and he felt like cursing me, calling me a "bastard, a fuck, a shit." As soon as he had uttered these words, he feared he would die as a result of having attacked me. He countered his hostility with isolated affectionate fantasies of me and my genitals, fantasies he said he did not believe. He feared "going too deep" and then became alarmed at the possibility of contracting hepatitis from a syringe. This idea, he said, was connected with a fear of being "stuck" by my penis.

During the next session, he again verbalized these fears and added that he was afraid he would be poisoned by swallowing ammonia water. He anticipated a return of a previously experienced dread of explosions. When I tried to show him that his fears were based on his daydreams, he became angry and said that I did not want to listen to his complaints. He added that he had feared that a policeman's horse would bite him if he did not feed it sugar, that he would be killed for neglecting the animal. His slip of "analyst" for "animal" enabled us to perceive his fury at me for neglecting him as his parents did. He reversed the situation by thinking the horse-animal-analyst would kill him. Continuing, he said that he felt like a girl and that his "behind itched." He told me that he had withheld his bowel movements for two days. Immediately, he poured forth anger at me and his father. What I said was "baloney" and he did not believe me. He had fears in order to evoke his parents' love. Then, five minutes before the close of the session, he informed me that he had dreamed that he was a girl with huge breasts. He also had had another dream, a wet dream, that had to do with his mother. I told him that he would rather have and talk of symptoms than deal with subjects like his wet dream; hence, he was telling me his fears of poisonous fluids rather than his fears of the wet dream fluid.

At our next meeting, Billy described a new fear, that of swallowing a button. He said he wanted to get away from home, to go to boarding school, but his mother refused and thus kept him from achieving this aim. After I had pointed out his attachment to his mother and his difficulty in separating from her, he described daydreams of touching Mrs. Y's breasts, fears of becoming ill if he touched his anus, and his need to "keep in" his bowel movements. He had had a bowel movement but had felt it was dangerous "to let it out."

At this point, I suggested that Billy's fears of dirt made it frightening for him to touch himself or to let things out. He was also afraid, I added, that if he touched himself, he would damage his penis and testicles. So he kept it all in and had symptoms instead. Billy's response to this interpretation was to say that he had thought of trying to let out his semen by having an ejaculation, but that he "could not let it out."

INITIAL DISCUSSION

I had best pause here and review what was occurring in the

analysis. Billy was afraid of being dirty or bad lest he be punished. This fear could be traced to his aunt's threats, which may have screened parental admonitions, and to his conflicts over toilet training. His phallic phase was colored by his anal fixation which had influenced the nature of his castration anxiety in relation to his masturbation. Despite his use of multiple defenses—including repression, denial, isolation, projection, displacement, reaction formation, and reversal—he did not succeed in allaying his anxiety sufficiently. As a consequence, he was dominated by obsessional fears and phobias.

The increase of anxiety at this point in Billy's life resulted from the intensification of his sexual and aggressive urges which normally accompany adolescence. In addition, the threat of terminating treatment led to an amplification of his sexual feelings toward the analyst, partly to counteract the hatred that the fantasied desertion engendered. More usually, a teenager's heightened sexuality impels him to seek genital discharge, but Billy found that he could not masturbate. Touching himself was dirty and could lead to his death. He had thought this during toilet training. For him, ejaculating semen was equivalent to letting his filthy bowel movement out, and this he could not do. In addition to all this, as we had learned earlier in the analysis, was his fear of injury to his genitals, both penis and testicles. He could be attacked, killed, and castrated by his father for sexual or hostile feelings. The bodily sensations of sexual excitement that he experienced included feelings that his genitals would explode and be destroyed. As we shall see, my suspicion that he was also afraid of the diminution of consciousness that occurs with sexual excitement and orgasm proved to be correct when he later confirmed my interpretation to that effect.

Billy was in a well-nigh intolerable position. He could not give vent to his urges to masturbate because for him masturbation was so dangerous. But without this means of discharge, his impulsive strivings grew in intensity, his forbidden sexual fantasies plagued him, and hence he had to struggle desperately against them. These fantasies appeared in his daydreams and, in more derivative form, in his symptomatology. Even thinly disguised oedipal and homosexual wishes burst into consciousness.

In the analytic sessions we were gradually coming to understand the nature of his impulses and the reasons for his fear of them. It was at this point that Billy was aware of his desire to masturbate and his simultaneous fear to do so.

CONTINUATION OF CLINICAL MATERIAL

Let us now return to the actual analytic hours.

After another terrified recitation of his fears, Billy said that he felt there was "something sexual" about them. They occurred, he thought, because he did not have an ejaculation. But when I agreed, he immediately negated this idea by saying that he had not known about masturbation until the previous year, when he had learned of it at a fraternity initiation. I acknowledged that he had not known the word, but reminded him that he had felt like carrying out the act years before. "How," Billy asked, "do people learn of masturbation? From each other?" This did occur, I agreed, but he also had learned of it from his body. His body told him to do it, but he, I said, was afraid because he pictured masturbation as dangerous and poisonous. Billy said he was surprised that touching the penis without ejaculation was also termed masturbation and then accused me of "leading him to masturbate." As doctors sometimes prescribe the wrong medicine, the directions I was giving him, he protested, might be wrong. He pointed his middle finger at me in an obscene gesture and then realized that he was angry at me. I told Billy that I had not said he should masturbate, but that I did think it might relieve him in certain ways. He was afraid, he responded, of injuring himself. Then, shortly before the close of the session, he remembered that he had had a wet dream.

I thought of Jim's [a friend's] mother. I felt her breast but not her nipple. I felt a rumbling, like a gun about to shoot off. I tried to hold it in, but could not.

When I commented that Billy's body was saying that it wanted to have an ejaculation, he replied that his fears increased at night. If he got better he would have to end the analysis, and he feared that he would kill himself.

The next day, after Billy had said that he was afraid of swallowing glass and dying, I attributed his fear of dying to a bodily desire to have an orgasm with the accompanying diminution or loss of consciousness. The idea that he could experience such a diminution alarmed him. "Now I won't have an ejaculation," he announced firmly. He was afraid of falling if he masturbated while standing at the toilet; and he could not masturbate in bed because masturbation was dirty! Then he recalled that when he had had the wet dream he had fallen into a deeper sleep after trying to hold in the semen.

Billy, in this same session, now talked of his fears at great length: fears of being bitten by a horse; fears of getting glass into his mouth. I said that probably these fears were related to daydreams of taking something into his mouth—breasts or a penis. He denied that such a thing could be true, but recalled that he did sometimes put his mouth close to his penis.

Billy's fears again dominated the first part of the next session. He was so frightened that he wanted to stay home from school. While in class he had felt a compulsion to move his hips in a motion that we agreed was sexual. He reminded himself that he had had a "boner" while talking to an old teacher with sagging breasts. An aunt of his, the one who had threatened him, had large breasts and she had once undressed before him. I explained to him that he had a need to masturbate and that masturbation included both the act and the thoughts connected with it. He tried to avoid the act and the thoughts, I said, but they appeared in both his fears and fantasies. On hearing this, Billy became more alarmed and again felt that I was urging him to masturbate. He wanted to have an extra session so that he would be protected against the dangerous consequences of masturbation.

I received a telephone call from Billy the next afternoon, a day on which he had no scheduled analytic hour. He told me that he had masturbated to ejaculation that morning. As he had expected, he had become dazed, but he had not anticipated that the feeling would continue as it had. He was afraid that he "would do something he did not want to do."

On his way to his next session, Billy noticed black smoke streaming from a chimney. This was dangerous and illegal and he would have liked to report it to the police, because smog killed people. He realized that the smoke stack reminded him of a penis and of his masturbation. He had, in fact, masturbated several times since his phone call to me. Initially, he had "done it" to attain relief, as I had said he might. He had masturbated in bed and had feared "making a mess." He had ejaculated in a short time and it had "felt like a drum roll." The next time he had masturbated for pleasure and, he said, "it *was* pleasant." As he talked, his fears returned, enabling me to show him how he was actually afraid of masturbation, but was deflecting his fears to other ideas. Calm again, he said that he had "thought of nothing" during masturbation. When I expressed skepticism, he said he had thought perhaps of a woman's breast in his mouth and had been upset lest he might bite it. "A nipple is like a penis," he said.

At this point Billy's parents had to leave town on urgent business and he decided to go with them. When he returned a week later, he reported with delight that his fears had disappeared and that he was able to masturbate without anxiety. As the analysis proceeded, this proved to be largely true. He experienced his fears in relatively minor form at times, but his crisis of intense terror was a thing of the past.

DISCUSSION II

To summarize briefly what was accomplished in this segment of the analysis: once Billy's inhibitions against masturbation decreased sufficiently so that he was able to reach an ejaculation, his pressing symptoms all but disappeared. The result was dramatic, but I should like to emphasize that I have described only a small portion of a relatively long analysis. For the most part, we worked hard and ploddingly as we analyzed Billy's characteristic defenses and gradually saw the drive derivatives against which he was defending. The usual prolonged working through processes and gradual changes were the predominant features of the analysis, not the more dramatic and sudden changes, the details of which I have here recounted.

Even in the few months described above, my technical interventions were restricted to preparation for interpretations and to interpretations proper. When I pointed out that Billy's fears were based on fantasy and not reality, he felt reassured, but my intent was to lay the groundwork for *interpretive* interventions aimed toward demonstrating that his fears arose from specific fantasies which, in turn, stemmed from specific wishes. My interpretations and his responses led to my awareness that Billy had been thinking of masturbating but felt that it was dangerous to "let things out." At this point, the picture became rather clear to me: I now suspected that unless Billy were able to masturbate, he would not attain relief from his symptoms. From that time on, I pointedly made comments about his fear of autoerotic activity and its consequences. Billy felt that I was urging him to masturbate when I made these remarks. Countertransferences could have stopped me from analyzing his fear of masturbatory activity at this point. Countertransferences could also have led to my urging him instead of analyzing him. Geleerd (1957) has noted that the "adolescent needs explanation and encouragement from the analyst to accept sexuality and aggression" (p. 273). In this case, interpretation sufficed. Later, we could understand that Billy's idea that I was suggesting he masturbate was an expression of his need to avoid responsibility for his own desires, of his need to be urged to defecate as he had been urged to do when he was being toilet trained; and, further, of his homosexual wishes to have me do something sexual to him. In this connection, a persistence of his symbiotic desires concurrent with his more mature heterosexual wishes is relevant. If I had actually advocated masturbation, the analysis of these defenses and fantasies would have been impeded and perhaps rendered impossible.

The result of Billy's ability to masturbate to a climax was quite remarkable. His obsessional fears and the phobias that he had previously been unable to control disappeared. When they occasionally reappeared, they were manageable. It would be valuable to discuss the determinants of this clinical change more carefully.

As I have suggested, Billy's increased need to masturbate arose from his phase-appropriate biological increase in drives. In addition, the threat of terminating the analysis and leaving home intensified his erotic transference and accentuated his need to masturbate in order to stem his hatred of the fantasied deserters who failed to protect him. His unconscious masturbation fantasies were those of union with mother, father, and analyst. He could orally incorporate breasts and penis, and thus keep close to, or be one with, potentially lost objects. Anal incorporation could serve the same purpose. These wishes and defenses had been under analytic scrutiny earlier and were further interpreted subsequent to the sessions which I have described.

Ordinarily during adolescence, the increased drives are partially dissipated through masturbation.[1] "Damming up" of sexual desires is thus kept to a minimum. This tension regulation prevents the development of the *physical* symptoms of sexual excitement and the *psychoneurotic* symptoms that are compromise expressions of id wishes and superego demands modified by the ego. The practice of masturbation also serves to prevent the acting out of the concomitant fantasies, such as Anna Freud (1949) described in younger children. I do not wish to imply that adolescents who masturbate do not develop symptoms or act out, merely to suggest that masturbation can serve as an alternative outlet. In this sense, masturbation can be an adaptive act that maintains autonomous ego functioning at a high level and prevents excessive tension and symptomatology.

In Billy's case, his castration anxiety prevented him from masturbating to orgasm. As I initially described, the severity of his castration anxiety and guilt was heightened by his anal fixations and further augmented by separation anxiety. Hence he could not attain the degree of ego mastery of sexual tension generally achieved in middle adolescence. Many of the symptoms that he had developed were clearly expressions of sexual fantasies. His fears of swallowing the button or glass, of being bitten by a horse, or of ingesting poison were manifestations of his desires to take a breast or penis into his mouth. His dread of being injured in a way that reminded him of anal intercourse and his belief that I would kill him reflected homosexual wishes. These wishes were also regressively disguised depictions of heterosexual (that is, positive oedipal) genital wishes. Punishment for the fantasied forbidden activity was integrated into the symptoms and the wishes were concealed by numerous defensive maneuvers.

Not only did Billy's fantasies appear in his symptomatology but so also did the wished for masturbatory act and its associated sensations. His fear of being poisoned by fluids was in part based on a wish to have fluid —semen—come out of his penis. His desire for an orgasm was also expressed in his fear of dying. In the orgastic experiences during wet dreams, he learned of the sensory changes before and during climaxes; he wished for the partial or complete unconsciousness (*la petite mort*) accompanying orgasm. Again, this wish represented punishment as well and hence appeared as the fear of death.

Billy experienced several other symptoms that were concomitants of sexual excitement. He was restless and irritable so that he easily became angry. As may be recalled, while at school he had strong urges to execute sexual pelvic movements. His concern that he might again develop a fear of explosions was, I believe, due to a beginning awareness of explosive feelings in the genitals and elsewhere. I also think that his hazy feelings, as if he were in a fog, were in part due to changes in the perceptual threshold that occur during sexual excitement, that is, to the diminished ability to perceive stimuli. Billy's hazy feelings were, I believe, similar to what Freud (1894) called *vertigo* in his description of neurasthenia.

Having discussed many of the determinants of Billy's symptomatology, I shall now consider the therapeutic process.

Prior to the time that the analysis of the masturbation inhibition became a central issue, interpretations dealt with the more general aspects of Billy's personality structure. His fear of separation from the analyst was related to his erotic and aggressive transference and its antecedents in early childhood when he had been left by his parents. We discussed his clinging attachment to his father, his mother, and his analyst, all of whom he felt were potential protectors who might neglect him. The conflict between his erotic and aggressive wishes and his punitive superego was analyzed and the relevant antecedents emerged. His regressive response to threatened separation was likewise analyzed.

This analytic work had some ameliorative effect, but of a temporary and intermittent nature only. The interpretations of the more specific conflicts regarding masturbation were more telling. These, of course, were both dependent on, and a continuation of, the previous analytic activity.

I pointed out Billy's desire to masturbate and the related fantasies which involved the analyst, his parents and substitutes. We discussed his superego's role in the creation of his dread of being injured or killed. His many displaced anxieties were linked to his fears of masturbation and to the associated affectionate and hostile wishes and fantasies. Other defenses were scrutinized as well. I also showed Billy how fears of bodily sensations, which were concomitants of sexual excitement and of the orgastic experience, contributed to his inability to masturbate.

Under the influence of these interpretations in the accepting, nonpunitive atmosphere of the analysis, Billy's superego was modified sufficiently to permit the masturbatory act and the attendant, derivative fantasies. Further, his ego became capable of tolerating the anticipated bodily reactions and the anxiety engendered by them. His anxiety was diminished and his reality testing was strengthened. Not only did the resolution of conflicts involving masturbation have a salutary effect, but the newly won ability to masturbate to ejaculation brought therapeutic benefits as well. An economic change had occurred. The discharge of sexual tension resulted in a decrease in drive pressure and with it, in fantasies, anxiety, and symptoms. Bodily sensations of sexual excitement were also diminished and this factor, along with his greater ability to tolerate such bodily states made for less anxiety.

As Billy and I could perceive later in the analysis, his ability to masturbate led to greater confidence in himself as an assertive male, to more open heterosexual fantasies and ultimately to the finding of a heterosexual, nonincestuous object.

"ACTUAL NEUROSIS" AND THE PHYSIOLOGICAL CONCOMITANTS OF SEXUAL EXCITEMENT

I have presented the foregoing clinical material primarily to illustrate an aspect of psychoanalytic treatment in adolescence. However, this material, itself, calls for an evaluation of the concept of the "actual neurosis," for those readers familiar with the early formulations of Freud must have been struck by what appears to have been the dramatic disappearance of an actual neurosis. In fact, although much of Billy's symptomatology was not the result of physical concomitants of sexual excitement, it might be valuable to tease out those components that were, so as to delineate such manifestations in this boy's case. Before doing this, however, a brief discussion of the concept "actual neurosis" will, I believe, provide a useful background. I would add that, in view of the disrepute to which this historical concept has fallen, it is probably preferable to employ the phrase "physiological concomitants of sexual excitement" rather than "actual neurosis" or "actual neurotic symptomatology."

Freud (1894) differentiated the psychoneuroses from the actual neuroses and included anxiety neurosis and neurasthenia in the latter category. The actual neuroses were conceived of as the result of failure to discharge sexual excitement appropriately with the consequent accumulation of toxic substances and the appearance of signs and symptoms of sexual tension. This state has been picturesquely but erroneously called one of dammed-up libido. According to Freud's classification, when the damming up results from complete abstinence or failure to achieve an orgasm, due to factors such as, for example, a husband's premature ejaculation, *anxiety neurosis* appears; but when there is incomplete discharge, as in excessive masturbation or nocturnal emissions, *neurasthenia*, including hypochondriasis, occurs. Psychoneurosis differs from an actual neurosis in that the symptoms of the former are psychologically determined, that is, they are symbolic expressions of wishes modified by compromise formation. Freud's first theory of anxiety as transformed libido is an extension of the concept of the actual neurosis, but he later reformulated his ideas about anxiety when he realized that it was a reaction to a danger situation from within or without.

Freud never abandoned the concept of the actual neurosis as he clearly states in *Inhibitions, Symptoms and Anxiety* (Freud, 1926). Although analysts have generally discarded this diagnosis, a few continue to employ it. Nunberg (1924), who maintains that such a state exists, says it is of theoretical rather than of practical value. Fink (1970) nevertheless has described analytic material that, he says, required an awareness of the actual neurosis for an appreciation of the relevant symptomatology. He drew on the observations of Masters and Johnson (1966) to strengthen his position. In his discussion of Fink's paper, Rangell (1968), restating his earlier formulation (1955), maintained that the actual neurosis does exist, and, even more recently, he affirmed that the actual neurosis is *indeed* the core of every psychoneurosis (1971). Rangell (1955) also stated that "damming up of instinctual energy is an economic-dynamic condition of unpleasure, and anxiety a specific reaction to the danger which this entails" (p. 397). He maintained that the resulting stimuli bring about a traumatic state which causes anxiety, and consequent psychoneurotic symptom formation.

Masters and Johnson have demonstrated that during sexual excitement people develop feelings which result from genital vasocongestion, swelling, and muscular contractions. Extragenital bodily changes occur as well. If an orgasm does not occur and excitement continues, more intense symptoms emerge. Freud (1894) anticipated this when he suggested that "somatic excitation is manifested as a pressure on the walls of the seminal vesicles, which are lined with nerve endings" (p. 108). These conduct impulses to the cerebral cortex with the ultimate development of a "psychic stimulus" (ibid., p. 108). The restlessness and irritability that Freud found in the actual neuroses are confirmed by Fink as well as Masters and Johnson, who also noted that they are relieved when the subject reaches a climax. As Glenn (1965, 1969) pointed out, the testicular swelling and vasocongestion known in common parlance as "blue balls," is a painful consequence of unsatisfied sexual excitement. Bornstein (1953) and Glenn (1965) mention penile discomfort in sexual tension. Fink mentions backache and gastric disorder as similar symptoms.

It is surely not a coincidence that several of the authors (Blos, 1962; Spiegel, 1958; Bernfeld, 1935) who state, unequivocally and without fuss, as if it were an obvious fact, that the actual neurotic symptoms exist, are analysts of adolescents.[2] Dealing with a patient population most likely to suffer from undischarged sexual excitement, they have observed the symptom manifestations of these in their teenage patients, as did Freud in his adult patients. Curiously, they have not offered clinical illustrations.

Blau (1952) has extended the concept of the actual neurosis to include traumatic neuroses and childhood behavior disorders where external circumstances create intolerable psychic conditions. He considers the physical concomitants of anxiety or anxiety equivalents to be actual neurotic symptoms and places psychosomatic disorders in this category. Friend (1956) suggests in a discussion of a paper by Blau and Hulse (1956) that the authors are not convincing "in their main thesis that 'actual' neuroses accounts for the syndrome, primary behavior disorders with conduct disturbance" (p. 118). The same statement can be made regarding the other conditions Blau (1952) describes, especially if Freud's original definitions are adhered to.

It is striking that the concept of the actual neurosis, developed in 1894, keeps cropping up, despite the fact that it is based on the prestructural conceptualization of the personality and was formulated at a time when a hydrodynamic model prevailed. I believe that this concept persists because contained within it is a kernel of truth, that is, the fact that there are physiological concomitants of' sexual excitement. Indeed, these concomitants may be insufficiently considered because of their association with the term "actual neurosis" and its discarded theoretical framework. But we should avoid discarding the valid components of this concept along with its incorrect and unsubstantiated aspects.

The following statements, based on clinical experience, can safely be made.

1. Physiological concomitants of sexual excitement exist. These may persist until the excitement ceases through orgasm or other means. Excitement and its manifestations may end with the passage of time, as Masters and Johnson (1966) have confirmed.

On the other hand, there is danger of confusing the empirical fact that certain symptoms persist during unrelieved sexual excitement with the hypothetical statement that dammed-up libido exists. This dubious theoretical formulation is based on the idea that psychic (libidinal) energy is equivalent to physical energy which accumulates in the peripheral organs.

2. Freud's classification, in which the actual neuroses are categorized as anxiety neurosis and neurasthenia, each with a different etiology, is unsupportable. Failure to achieve sexual release either completely or incompletely can result in a variety of symptoms: excessive tension, explosive feelings, restlessness, altered ego states, backache, genital discomfort and swelling, and so forth.

3. The anxiety that follows sexual excitement is not transformed libido; it is the ego's reaction to a danger situation. Organisms react with the same manifestations to other types of internal or external danger.

4. The danger situation may at times be traumatic in that it may be beyond the ego's capacity to contain the excessive internal stimulation involved in the unrelieved sexual excitement. But it need not on other occasions be traumatic in this strict sense of the term (Furst, 1967). The erotic feelings may come in conflict with the superego or ego with resultant anxiety. Whether the individual will experience the physical concomitants of sexual excitement as symptoms will depend on the magnitude of the physical changes and resultant sensations, on the individual's ability to recognize their origin, and on his tolerance of sexual excitement.

5. The physiological concomitants may be intertwined with psychoneurotic symptomatology. Freud recognized this when he stated that actual neurotic and psychoneurotic symptoms were interrelated. The physiological concomitants may call forth anxiety and consequent defensive activity with resultant symptomatology, as we have seen in the clinical material presented in this paper. These concomitants may unconsciously be given special meaning by the individual, as, for example, when a woman's low

backache, a result of uterine congestion, comes to represent the punishment for sexual or aggressive wishes. Or, as demonstrated by Heiman (1963) and Glenn (1965), the visceral sensations may play a determining role in the development of fantasies, self-representations, and symbols.

6. Freud's belief that toxic substances cause the physiological concomitants of sexual excitement has not been confirmed. Aside from the fact that it is strange to consider such chemicals as toxins even if they cause symptoms, such specific substances have not been found. A possible exception is mentioned by Heiman (1963) who describes a pituitary hormone released when the breasts are stimulated. Of course, the physical changes during sexual excitement are mediated by the autonomic nervous system.

It is because of the deficiencies inherent in and associated with Freud's concept of the actual neurosis that I have suggested that this term should be abandoned. By the same token, I have suggested that the concept of *physiological concomitants of sexual excitement* should be maintained, because it is this concept which constitutes the core of truth in Freud's use of the term "actual neurosis."

I return now to Billy in order to reevaluate which of his symptoms were, at least in part, physiological concomitants of sexual excitement. I have already mentioned his restlessness, irritability, pelvic movements, his explosive feelings, and his hazy feelings as results of sexual excitement.

I have also suggested that the confusing bodily sensations during prolonged sexual excitation can lead to preoccupation with or worry about the body, that is, to hypochondriasis. In such cases, there can be a complication in that displacement of cathexis from the genitals to other areas or the body as a whole occurs. Billy was also concerned about the state of his penis and testicles and this concern then spread by displacement to other parts of his body which he repeatedly scanned for signs of injury. Freud (1894) stated that hypochondriasis occurs as part of the clinical picture of neurasthenia which is due to incomplete discharge, such as through nocturnal emission with no other relief. Wet dreams were indeed Billy's only means of ejaculation.

In view of the similarity between Billy's state of haziness on the one hand, and depersonalization and other altered states of consciousness on the other hand, we may postulate that such states, especially when they occur transiently in adolescence, may be built on a base comprised of the sensations or altered thresholds of perception due to sexual excitement. Of course, other contributing factors play a role as well. Freud (1909), Stamm (1962), and Dickes (1965), among others, have discussed defensive and regressive factors in altered ego states. Quite possibly Billy's fear of insanity, which I have not discussed in this clinical report, and which is commonly thought by adolescents to be causally linked to masturbation, was also determined by his experience of these altered states of consciousness during sexual excitement and following orgasm. This fear of insanity, then, can result from causes other than the more generally observed mechanism, that is, the displacement of castration anxiety from the genitals to the brain.

Now, while I considered Billy's restlessness, irritability, hypochondriasis, and hazy feelings to be due, in part, to sexual excitement, this was not the case in respect to his anxiety. Rather, his extreme anxiety was attributable to the fact that, under the influence of his superego, his ego perceived the phase specific, increased drive pressure as dangerous. His failure to achieve discharge was the consequence of his fear of sexual excitement and the effects of orgasm. In snowball fashion, the intensification of Billy's anxiety was commensurate with the increase of his sexual excitement and associated bodily sensations. Psychoneurotic symptoms, in turn, were amplified as defenses against anxiety, and drives were mobilized.

From the economic viewpoint, we must consider the appearance of the concomitants of sexual excitement as a narcissistic phenomenon. Narcissism is defined (Freud, 1914; Jacobson,

1964; Bing et al., 1959) as libidinal cathexis of the self-representation or, as is especially pertinent here, the self. Jacobson (1964) and Bing et al. (1959) have suggested that the body, itself, is cathected in infancy during the undifferentiated phase preceding the formation of self and object representations. In adolescence, the increased libidinal and aggressive cathexis of the parents is forbidden and dangerous. Attempts to withdraw cathexis from these object representations eventuate in increased cathexis of the self (including the body) or its representation; the teenager becomes more narcissistic.

As we have seen in Billy's analysis, the cathectic shifts in adolescence need not be complete. Indeed they never are. Oedipal fantasies burst forth and may be defended against by regression to pre-oedipal attachments. Billy had not yet succeeded in finding new objects. As I have indicated, at a later phase he was to achieve this.

NOTES

[1]In this paper, I will not discuss the related question of attaining relief through heterosexual activity.

[2]See also Reich (1951) and Fenichel (1945).

BIBLIOGRAPHY

Arlow, J.A. 1953. Masturbation and symptom formation. *Journal of the American Psychoanalytic Association* 1:45-58.

Bernfeld, S. 1935. On simple male adolescence. *Zeitschrift für Psychoanalytische Pedagogik* 9:360-79. Translated in *Seminars in psychiatry* 1:113-26.

Bing, J.F., McLaughlin, F., and Marburg, R. 1959. The metapsychology of narcissism. *Psychoanalytic Study of the Child* 14:9-28.

Blau, A. 1952. In support of Freud's syndrome of "actual" anxiety neurosis. *International Journal of Psycho-Analysis* 33:363-72.

Blau, A., and Hulse, W.C. 1956. Anxiety ("actual") neuroses as a cause of behavior disorders in children. *American Journal of Orthopsychiatry* 26:108-14.

Blos, P. 1962. *On adolescence*. New York: Free Press of Glencoe.

Bornstein, B. 1953. Masturbation in the latency period. *Psychoanalytic Study of the Child* 8:65-78.

Dickes, R. 1965. The defensive function of an altered state of consciousness: A hypnoid state. *Journal of the American Psychoanalytic Association* 13:356-403.

Fenichel. O. 1945. *The psychoanalytic theory of the neurosis*. New York: W. W. Norton.

Fink, P.J. 1970. Correlations between "actual" neurosis and the work of Masters and Johnson. *Psychoanalytic Quarterly* 39:38-51.

Freud, A. 1949. Certain types and stages of social maladjustment. In *Searchlights on delinquency*, ed. K.R. Eissler. New York: International Universities Press.

———. 1958. Adolescence. *Psychoanalytic Study of the Child* 13:255-78.

Freud, S. 1895. On the grounds for detaching a particular syndrome from neurasthenia under the description "anxiety neurosis." *Standard edition*, vol. 3. London: Hogarth Press.

———. 1909*a*. Some general remarks on hysterical attacks. *Standard edition*, vol. 9. London: Hogarth Press.

———. 1909*b*. Analysis of a phobia in a five-year-old boy. *Standard edition*, vol. 10. London: Hogarth Press.

———. 1914. On narcissism: An introduction. *Standard edition*, vol. 14. London: Hogarth Press.

———. 1926. Inhibitions, symptoms and anxiety. *Standard edition*, vol. 20. London: Hogarth Press.

Friend, M.R. 1956. Discussion of Blau and Hulse's "Anxiety ('actual') neuroses as a cause of behavior disorders in children." *American Journal of Orthopsychiatry* 26:114-18.

Furst, S.S., ed. 1967. *Psychic trauma*. New York: Basic Books.

Geleerd, E.R. 1957. Some aspects of psychoanalytic technique in adolescence. *Psychoanalytic Study of the Child* 12:263-83.

Glenn, J. 1965. Sensory determinants of the symbol *three*. *Journal of the American Psychoanalytic Association* 13:422-34.

———. 1969. Testicular and scrotal masturbation. *International Journal of Psycho-Analysis* 50:353-62.

Heiman, M. 1963. Sexual response in women: A correlation of physiological findings with psychoanalytic concepts. *Journal of the American Psychoanalytic Association* 11:360-85.

Jacobson, E. 1964. *The self and the object world*. New York: International Universities Press.

Masters, W.H., and Johnson, V.E. 1966. *Human sexual response*. Boston: Little, Brown.

Nunberg, H. 1924. States of depersonalization in the light of the libido theory. In *Practice and theory of psychoanalysis*, vol. 1. New York: International Universities Press, 1948.

Rangell, L. 1955. On the psychoanalytic theory of anxiety: A statement of a unitary theory. *Journal of the American Psychoanalytic Association* 3:389-414.

———. 1968a. Discussion of Fink's "Correlations between 'actual' neurosis and the work of Masters and Johnson" at American Psychoanalytic Association meetings, May 1968.

———. 1968b. A further attempt to resolve the "problem of anxiety." *Journal of the American Psychoanalytic Association* 16:371-404.

———. 1971. Personal communication.

Reich, A. 1951. The discussion of 1912 on masturbation and our present views. *Psychoanalytic Study of the Child* 6:80-94.

Spiegel, L.A. 1951. A review of contributions to a psychoanalytic theory of adolescence: Individual aspects. *Psychoanalytic Study of the Child* 6:375-93.

———. 1958. Comments on the psychoanalytic psychology of adolescence. *Psychoanalytic Study of the Child* 13:296-308.

Stamm, J.L. 1962. Altered ego states allied to depersonalization. *Journal of the American Psychoanalytic Association* 10:762-83.

Episodes of Severe Ego Regression in the Course of an Adolescent Analysis

Selma Kramer, M.D. *Philadelphia*

INTRODUCTION

As my contribution to this book, I have selected material from two separate episodes of delusional thinking, which occurred in the course of a long analysis of an adolescent boy. My purpose in doing this is to add this clinical material to that of others so that the question of analyzability of adolescents may be considered anew. Notable in this case, and requisite for the analysis, was the presence of a solid therapeutic relationship. Donald trusted me enough to tell me of his delusions and to continue analyzing them even when, as in the second episode, I was woven into the delusional structure.

Donald was in analysis from 15 to 21 years of age. The analysis brought to light the many liabilities which taxed this boy's ego and mitigated against his growing up. Among these liabilities were his mother's paranoid psychosis; the taking over by his father of certain mothering functions early in Donald's life; extremely precocious puberty (at 9-1/2 years); and a severe, disfiguring pustular acne. It is significant that at 10 Donald had a well-defined obsessive-compulsive neurosis which collapsed with the upsurge of sexual and aggressive drives as adolescence proceeded. These topics will come into this paper as the highlights of the analysis are covered, but the main focus will be on the episodes of paranoid ideation. The first occurred early in the analysis, within the first year, and the second, about midway through.

In each instance, I had to consider whether the analysis, itself, might endanger this boy's very fragile ego, which evidenced considerable distortion of reality testing. This danger was weighed against positive factors such as the position of other ego functions and the strength of the therapeutic relationship. In each case, when this specific regression to psychotic thinking occurred, Donald was evidencing improved tolerance for anxiety in other areas, and generally increased ego strength. Also, the therapeutic relationship had developed to the point where Donald could ally his observing ego with the investigative function of the analyst. Another significant factor was that Donald looked to psychoanalysis for relief from the intense emotional pain he experienced prior to analysis. As Geleerd (1957) stated: "Treatment [of adolescents] is more easily accepted by youngsters whose neuroses cause disturbances that are accompanied by suffering which cannot be denied." Prior to starting analysis, anxiety made it almost impossible for Donald to attend school. He had insomnia, fearsome outbursts of temper, severe acne which contributed to his self-contempt, and frequent periods of depression.

PART I: PREFACE TO THE ANALYSIS

Donald was referred to me at the age of 10 for what his parents euphemistically called his "habits," which had begun a few months prior to the referral. These "habits" were compulsions which he had to repeat for a multiple of four, often up to sixty-four times; they usually involved his sitting down and then rising from a chair. If interrupted, Donald became frantic and angry, saying that if he did not complete the series of actions he would turn into a "brat" or a "liar" or a "cheater." Otherwise, his parents felt that Donald was a good, well-behaved boy who did well in school but had very few friends. After Donald had insisted on remaining out of doors in a thunderstorm in order to comply with his rituals, his parents had become alarmed and had consulted their family doctor who had then referred them to me.

His mother's main concern with Donald's symptoms was that the neighbors would tell everybody that he was insane. Mrs. Y felt that the neighbors gossiped about the family and that they were deliberately cutting to her, often pretending not to see her when she passed them. Further consultation with Mrs. Y revealed that she was suffering from a paranoid psychosis. As if in constant expectation of hostility, she wore a habitual, sarcastic sneer; and she told me that she had definite proof that others were talking about her.

Mrs. Y gave most of Donald's history, focusing first, however, on her own unhappy childhood. Mrs. Y felt that she was "the runt of the litter," unwanted because she was "only a girl." She dropped out of school when she was 14 because she believed that the teachers were deliberately cruel and that the other children were ridiculing her. She spent most of her adolescence and young adulthood at home, working sporadically until, at 26, she married. For the first three years of the marriage, the Y's lived with Mrs. Y's parents.

Mrs. Y wanted children and was upset by an infertility problem, although she felt that Mr. Y's low sperm count absolved her from blame. After two years of Mr. Y's treatment (and within two months of moving from her parents' home), Mrs. Y became pregnant. She spotted during early pregnancy and, at the end, developed toxemia. After three episodes of false labor, Donald was born following a prolonged, difficult labor. His mother was depressed for about six months, but, nonetheless, functioned. She was never again able to become pregnant. She had many gynecological complaints which finally resulted in a hysterectomy when Donald was 18.

Mrs. Y described Donald as having been a pleasant, easily managed infant, who ate well, adjusted to a rigid feeding schedule, and also slept well. Toilet training was initiated when he was less than 1 year old and was completed at 1-1/2 years. His general health was good except for multiple allergies. Mrs. Y mentioned pointedly, and without pride, that Donald had always been large for his age. At the time of this conference, when Donald was 10, the Y's revealed that they had been taking him to a dermatologist since the age of 8-1/2 in order to prevent his developing acne which each parent had had to a severe degree during mid-adolescence. At this time, the Y's felt that the dermatologist's advice was good since Donald indeed did not have acne. They did not tell me what this advice was.

In another interview, I asked Mrs. Y to tell me more about her feelings concerning Donald's height, since it had been obvious to me that she was uncomfortable about this. She said that when Donald was 3, he was as tall as most 5-year-olds, so that whenever the children in the neighborhood had engaged in any mischief, Donald, of course, had been singled out as the ringleader. Also, when he was 3, a neighbor had complained that Donald had hurt her child. At first, Mrs. Y could not believe this. She had felt that Donald was being "picked on" by the neighbors as she had been "picked on" when she was a child. However, when a second neighbor made a similar complaint, Mrs. Y panicked and furiously spanked Donald lest he become "a dangerous tough." Soon after this last incident, the family moved, presumably to buy a house large enough to share with Mrs. Y's parents. When I asked whether they had moved because of Donald's fight, Mrs. Y said: "Well, you know how it is when a child gets a bad reputation. It sticks with him for the rest of his life."

Donald seemed saddened by the move and thereafter rarely went out to play. Mrs. Y recognized that Donald may have connected outdoor play with the spanking he had received for his show of aggression. She revealed, however, that she was more comfortable with Donald in the house because, as she said, "When boys grow up they do dangerous things." When Donald was in latency, his mother did not encourage him to roller skate and she forbade bicycling as too dangerous. Compliantly, Donald turned to books and spent most of his time indoors.

In a separate interview, Mr. Y described the marriage as a good one, adding that troubles arose only when he tried to protect Donald from Mrs. Y's overstrictness. He mentioned that his wife had "no touching" prohibitions which she enforced on Donald and even on her husband. For example, freshly ironed shirts or curtains might not be touched, and no one was allowed to use the dining room furniture. (In the course of the analysis, Donald revealed that Mrs. Y did not permit either Mr. Y or Donald to sit on the living room sofa, insisting that they must sit on the floor to watch television.)

Mr. Y also disclosed that, when Donald was 2 months old, Mrs. Y had expressed the thought that Donald was "strange" and different from other children for she had felt that he looked at her "funny." When he was 4 or 5 years old, she said that Donald was too emotional and giggly. She now felt that Donald's present symptoms were evidence that she had been "right all along." The referring physician, who had known Donald all his life, said that Donald had been in no way atypical as an infant or as a young child.

Mr. Y described his own childhood as idyllic. He made no mention whatsoever of his mother; instead, he focused on his good fortune in having had an extremely close relationship with his own father. In adolescence and young adulthood, Mr. Y continued to maintain an interest in athletics, which had begun in childhood play with his father, by playing baseball with his old buddies each weekend. Mr. Y's utopian existence was destroyed at 23, when his father remarried after having been a widower for about a year. Crushed, Mr. Y felt that he could never again trust his father nor could he ever forgive him. However, he told me that he was sure that his father must have married for companionship and certainly not for sex. The two men were estranged and Mr. Y's father died suddenly three years later. Thereafter, Mr. Y felt lonely and depressed. At 26, he dated for the first time, and three months later he married.

Mr. Y was eager to have sons, wishing to repeat the happy elements of his own father-son relationship. Donald, however, did not respond well to his father's attempts to make a ballplayer of him. He did not even seem to appreciate his father's efforts to organize the neighborhood children so that Donald might have friends. Often Mr. Y would find himself playing with the other children while Donald sulked at home.

Mr. Y also described Donald as being rather isolated, with few friends; Mr. Y could not understand this contrast to his own adolescent pleasure with friends. Even so, he felt that Donald should not be pushed to socialize more and he emphasized the fact that he was glad to have his son close to home.

Serious pathology was evident in both parents. Mrs. Y revealed her own poor self-concept which was extended to include Donald; and the many obsessive-compulsive phenomena which controlled her and which, in turn, she used to control her husband and son. Her paranoia was revealed by her ideas of reference about the neighbors. Mr. Y was an extremely passive, effeminate man. The fact that Mr. Y mothered Donald, which had been suggested in the history, was borne out later when Donald's conflicts about homosexuality came into the analysis.

Arrangements were made to evaluate Donald, but the appointments were broken. Donald refused to come. I met with the parents a number of times in order to help them deal with Donald's resistance. When it became apparent that their own resistances were insurmountable, I discontinued efforts to see Donald. I felt that even if they could get themselves to bring Donald to me, I could not count on their cooperation to carry out a treatment plan for their son.

PART II: THE ANALYSIS

Five years later, when Donald was 15, I was asked to see him on an emergency basis. The complaint was of severe temper tantrums which had started six months before and which were now recurring with increasing severity and frequency. On the day before this frantic call, and at the culmination of a rage, Donald had pulled a banister from the wall and had smashed it to pieces. The parents were frightened and felt that Donald must really be crazy. They were terrified by his outbursts and feared his destructive strength. They were certain that they could not control this powerful, tall, adolescent son.

Donald came most willingly for exploratory appointments. He was an extremely tall, almost cadaverously thin 15-year-old with severe pustular acne. He spoke under such pressure that he almost stammered as he told me that he was terrified of his rages and of his inability to control his temper; and he pleaded with me to help him.

It was impossible for me not to be aware of the intense suffering of this boy. Yet, from the beginning, I felt that it would be necessary to avoid being drawn into the arena of his panic as he seemed to wish me to be. The previous contact with his parents had suggested the extent to which Donald received secondary gain from their responses when he exhibited himself as sick or troubled.

Rather than focusing on Donald's affect, I asked him to tell me about his tantrums. Donald described his outbursts as arising from "nothing at all" and then accelerating until they reached fearful heights. He said ruefully that he had known he had "this badness" in himself when his parents had consulted me for his "habits" five years ago. When I asked him why he had refused to come to see me at that time, Donald said wearily: "All they had to do was to insist on my seeing you, but they never insisted. I said 'no' and they said 'okay.' "

During exploratory appointments, Donald complained a great deal about schoolwork, which he had previously found easy. Now in the tenth grade, his marks had slipped so that he required help from his father each night. Donald approached every day with great panic, fearing school and hating each moment of it. Occasionally he feigned illness, but he felt guilty when he lied to miss school. He felt truly ill sometimes because of his severe allergies and, in the hay fever season, he could scarcely breathe. Donald acknowledged, however, that although he had had hay fever most of his life, the symptoms had never been sufficiently severe to keep him at home. At times, Donald complained about the teachers and the other students, expressing some vague remarks about their unfriendliness. However, in the early months of our contact, Donald concentrated on two problems: his temper outbursts and his problem in maintaining his standing in school. He was almost pathetically eager to come and describe to me his inability to concentrate and his great difficulty in finishing homework.

I arranged to see Donald four times a week as I felt that psychoanalysis was indicated for this boy. I did not think that anything less intensive could help him. The temper tantrums alone were, of course, of great concern to his parents and to Donald, and represented his ego's inability to handle impulses which were so overwhelming. Since adolescents do have temper tantrums, I did not feel that the tantrums alone would have necessitated analysis. However, there were other problems of adolescent life. His social life was very poor; he was becoming a recluse. It was more and more difficult for him to attend school and it was evident that he had a manifest separation problem. In addition, he found it extremely hard to cope with the ordinary responsibilities of school. This factor was indicated by his report card on which instead of his usual A's and high B's he was now getting C's and D's.

The early months of analysis revealed that Donald's need for his father's help had led Mr. Y to change his entire work schedule. A professional person, accustomed to working evenings, Mr. Y stayed home to go over Donald's work. Donald was panicked by each assignment and rendered utterly distraught by examinations.

His father outlined Donald's work with him and even wrote his compositions.

Donald began to try to alarm me, too, with the magnitude of his work and described the impossibility of pleasing the teachers who were out to get him. During one such episode, after four months of analysis, Donald dashed into the office sweating, his face flushed. He immediately told me that it was impossible for him to get his schoolwork done, and furthermore, coming to see me was not helping, but, in fact, was hindering him, since his appointments consumed two hours of his day. I told Donald that he seemed to feel that I was not helping him in the way he thought I should. He responded with anger and told me that he knew I did not take his school problems seriously enough. I remained so calm, he said, that he knew I did not care. I commented: "So, to show that I care about your school problems, I should become alarmed." Donald thought for a moment and said: "That's what my father does. He gets very excited and cancels his appointments with his clients; and he paces up and down awhile and then he works with me until my work is done." After some silence, Donald said he knew that he wanted me to get upset and that he got angry when I did not do so. But, at the same time, he said, he was relieved that I "kept my cool."

Of course, Donald's attempts to convince me of his need for help continued for a period of time. About two weeks after the episode described above, Donald brought his homework assignment to the office.

He said: "Look at this stuff. You can't convince me in a million years that I can do it. I know you feel I should do it without my father's help." (I had made no such comment to Donald but our discussions of his homework practices were making him aware of his excessive dependence upon his father.)

Donald proceeded to read each assignment and to ask me: "How would you do this problem?" or "Just tell me how you'd answer this question." I remained silent and as Donald began to flip through his textbooks and notes, he found that he had the necessary information and skills readily available. He was pleased but still angry as he said: "Gee, you must think I'm dumb!"

I commented that for weeks Donald had tried to convince me that he was dumb, but that today he seemed to have very mixed feelings when he found out that he was not dumb at all. Donald's retort was to pick up the word *today* and to say that maybe the homework was not so hard today, but there was no guarantee that it would not be too hard for him to do alone tomorrow or the next day. Since he knew I would not do it for him, he said, he would just have to go on having his father help him.

I then returned to his ambivalence about being "smart or dumb" with me, commenting he seemed so afraid that if he recognized he was smart it would interfere with his relationship with his father. He said his father liked to help him. In fact, his father sounded pleased and important when he called to cancel appointments with clients. He explained to them that his son needed his help with schoolwork.

Soon after Donald began to work on his own, I received an agitated and angry phone call from Mr. Y, complaining that I was taking his son from him, for Donald had actually refused his father's help. On the phone, I calmed Mr. Y by indicating that Donald was not rejecting him as a father, but that it was necessary for Donald to do more of his own work if school were not to be so menacing to him.

Donald's need to act "dumb" for his father and to try to impress me with his ineptness was the forerunner of later material which evidenced his need to be innocent, "dumb," asexual, or castrated. This allowed him to maintain erotic closeness to his father without guilt, a mechanism similar to the pseudo-imbecility so well described by Mahler (1942). "It is known . . . that the intellectual restriction is often used to disguise aggression in order to escape retaliation. Pseudo-stupidity, in addition, has been described as a display of castration to escape literal fear of castration and the loss of a loved object" (p. 153).

The analysis, now of fifteen months' duration, made Donald

conscious of the fact that he felt obliged to be the dependent little boy who could not function without his father's closeness. Donald recognized the two sides of his problem, namely that his father fostered his dependency and that Donald liked the attention he received from his father, for it made him feel loved. Donald angrily blamed me for trying to separate him from his father. As if to prove that he still needed his father's help, Donald failed two tests. At home he had a severe temper tantrum, the only one since treatment had begun. His parents called to report that he had banged on the basement walls shouting obscenities for approximately an hour.

Donald was extremely upset at his next appointment. When he strode in, he announced that he was angry with me because I was destroying the close relationship with his father which he so much needed. As an afterthought, he mentioned the tantrum of the previous night and added that analysis was not helping him if he still had tantrums.

I said that I felt the two issues, Donald's feeling that I was destroying the relationship with his father, and the temper tantrum, were connected. Donald started out angrily, "Connections, that's all you talk about!" Then he recalled having been very guilty the previous night when he had told his father that he could write a composition by himself. His father had seemed hurt and disappointed and had said, "I may as well see a client." Donald had begun to write his paper but had found that the ideas he had already organized in his mind "just wouldn't come out." He had become more and more upset and had begun to throw his books around his room. Soon he had gone to the basement and had shouted and pounded on the wall. Donald's mother had become agitated and had called her husband who had come home immediately. His father had said: "This boy certainly needs to continue treatment." Donald told me that he had been relieved when his father had said that.

Donald realized, therefore, that part of the motivation for the tantrum arose from his guilt over hurting and disappointing his father by no longer using his help with school work. At the same time, it served the purpose of making certain that his parents would keep him in analysis. During this session, Donald blurted out suddenly that he had a thought that he could not understand. Blushing and stammering, he said that maybe he had to keep his father at home at night. Then, as if he had proceeded too far and too fast, Donald became exceedingly tense and denied that there was any sense in such a stupid thought, although I might think otherwise.

At this time, Donald came close to becoming aware of his use of pseudo-stupidity as a means of staying close to his father, without guilt, until his homosexual panics occurred which then culminated in the violent temper outbursts.

This aspect of Donald's problems is similar to the more pervasive pseudo-stupidity described by Marjorie P. Sprince (1967). In describing her case, Sprince says: "Ivan's pseudo-stupidity was, at the deep level, a response to his passive homosexual wishes. By his stupid behavior, he repeatedly reassured his father of the continuation of the union and of the fact that the inferior qualities of the union remained rested in himself."

The emergence of this relatively undefended material resulted in greatly increased anxiety. There was a deflection of focus, resulting in the emergence of extremely paranoid-like material about his neighbors and mine.

First Episode of Paranoid Thinking

Donald was certain that his neighbors hated him and ignored him. He described numerous instances in which he felt snubbed or ridiculed and said that his neighbors were very "stuck-up" people who must consider him "crazy after hearing him shout so much." Donald was now able to reveal that he always shouted close up against the wall that separated the two houses. He recognized that he did this when he was furious at his mother and wanted to embarrass her, but he firmly believed, along with his mother, that the neighbors were guilty of listening at the walls. Donald said repeatedly that they deliberately sneered at him and his mother.

This material had such an extremely paranoid flavor that I was very concerned about Donald's mental condition. Yet at this time, when there was specific regression to psychotic or to psychotic-like thinking, Donald was evidencing satisfactory ego strength in other areas. The therapeutic alliance had developed to a point where Donald could usually ally his observing ego with the investigative function of the analyst. By the time Donald had reported the episode of the tantrum and had told me of his ideas of reference, he was showing increased tolerance for anxiety. He was able to attend school regularly and to do work on his own, and he was beginning to make a few friends. Donald was cooperative because he looked to psychoanalysis as the one source of relief from his fear of losing control, and from the great emotional pain that he experienced when he felt himself to be the object of his neighbors' ridicule and disdain. However, I judged that, at this point in analysis, Donald could not handle the conscious knowledge of the homosexual pull toward his father nor the extent of his mother's illness. Consequently, I dealt with this material as I would any other disclosure of a patient, cautiously exploring it with him and encouraging him to associate to it.

In keeping with this, I told Donald that it was important that we try to understand his expectations that his neighbors would dislike him. Donald revealed that he felt suspicious about my neighbors also. When he saw my next-door neighbor raking her lawn, he felt that she looked at him with suspicion and dislike. Since she was often out of doors at the time of his appointment, he felt that she must be there because she wondered why I was seeing such a disturbed boy. (In point of fact, my next-door neighbor was out of doors much of the time.)

The emergence of this material in the transference gave me the opportunity to explore Donald's ideas of reference within the framework of the analysis. When I commented: "You must be very worried about what my neighbor thinks of you if you feel she is suspicious of you and dislikes you," Donald said she looked like "a busybody" and "a gossip" who must wonder how crazy he was and also must think he was "a slob" and even ugly. Donald and I had previously spoken of his fear that coming for analysis must mean that he was crazy. When I referred to this conversation, Donald said that my neighbor would think that he was crazy primarily because of the way he looked. He went on to say that when he and his mother had argued recently about the way he dressed, his mother had shouted, "I don't know how Dr. Kramer can stand to look at you."

Donald went on to recall that, when he was very young, he was always admonished by his mother to be on his good behavior at family gatherings lest he stand out as bad in contrast to his good cousins. He was so awed and inhibited in the presence of company that he would become immobilized. At that point, his mother would whisper loudly that he should relax and play, which he could never do. Although Donald's mother always selected his clothes, she berated him for looking poorly dressed while his cousins wore their clothes better, were less clumsy, and even had nicer smiles. Donald said with genuine pain that his mother's criticism had become worse since his acne had developed.

I returned to Donald's mention of his mother's statement, "I don't know how Dr. Kramer can stand to look at you," and I added that this was Donald's concern too. Donald said that sometimes when I smiled he suspected me of smiling sarcastically as his mother often did. He could not believe that I was not repelled by his pimples or bothered by his height. I told Donald that the things that he was particularly concerned about right now centered around the evidence of his adolescent development. He knew from our previous discussions that his skin problem was connected with his sexual maturation and that his height had to do with his skeletal growth. Donald picked this up and remembered how difficult life had been for him because he had reached puberty at 9-1/2. His growth spurt had begun years before that of his peers. He described how awful it was to be so hairy and to need a deodorant. He wondered whether he would ever stop growing and recalled now a thought which he had not remembered to tell me. Donald said with hesitancy and discomfort: "I thought these dirty things, like the acne and the B.O., were my fault because I had done something bad." Donald could not go on with this material in spite of my attempts to help him.

I realized that Donald was very close to discussing masturbation. His anxiety was mounting to such a point, however, that I felt I should continue to focus on Donald's conflicts of very early puberty, which were relatively more ego-syntonic, rather than focus on his immediate masturbation problem. I commented, therefore, that now we could understand the symptoms that he had originally been referred for, the "habits" which he had said were necessary to keep him from being bad. To this, he added that he had tried so hard to stop what he could not control in himself—the sudden spurt of growth, the early sexual development, and his troublesome fantasies. Donald now associated to his feeling that girls were "bitches" whom he could not trust. I referred here to the transference implications by saying: "You must wonder whether you can trust me to accept you and your fantasies when they continue to be distasteful and upsetting." Donald replied that he could not see this in terms of his feelings about me. He added that he envied his friends who were dating. When he was around girls, he found it impossible to do anything but ward them off with sarcasm and rough speech. (Later in the analysis, Donald described a recurrent masturbation fantasy in which a pretty but mean girl tried to win him while he became increasingly angry until, at the point of ejaculation, he swore vile words at her.)

This material was followed by a regressive pull to his father. Donald recalled his father's comforting warmth when he was little or sick. Donald said ruefully that he was not getting much comfort from his father anymore and that he missed this, although he knew he should not. Donald continued to idealize his father, describing him as a "real" intellectual, but a kind one, not cold as some intellectuals were. Donald went on to say that there were times when it was apparent that his father did not know as much as he. This changed their relationship and Donald was not sure that his father liked the change. For the most part, however, Donald's overidealization of his father continued. The juxtaposition of his expressed fury at the girl, who was a mean, seductive "bitch" whom he could not trust, with the material in which he over-idealized his father shows an exaggeration of the normal development idealization of the father described by Mahler (1966) in her discussion of Greenacre's paper, *Problems of Overidealization of the Analyst and Analysis*. Mahler states:

- The father becomes a love object at a point at which the toddler's dangerous disillusionment with a now separate mother, and his realization of his own relative helplessness have been combining to produce a regressive pull toward re-engulfment in the earlier mother-child symbiosis. The stimulation and promotion of new experiences, which partial identification with the father at this point facilitates, is on a higher, less *instinctually contaminated* level than the toddler had originally *ever* attained with the 'need-satisfying mother'. The mother could not possibly alleviate all the 'bad' inner and outer experiences that the small infant's everyday life is bound to contain, and which the mother is expected to magically relieve or ward off.

  The father—the 'knight in shining armour'—is an uncontaminated heroic figure on whose image the longed-for fantasied, still relatively aggrandized self-image can be projected (p. 637).

The process which Mahler describes took place in an exaggerated form in Donald's early life. There was much more than the normal disillusionment with the "need-satisfying mother" since his mother was, in fact, a disturbed, dissatisfied woman who projected her own feelings of inadequacy and unacceptability onto Donald and treated him with disdain and overprotection. His father, in certain ways, was a "knight in shining armour" and remained, for too long a time in Donald's life, a heroic figure. Donald was not able to see his father realistically until quite late in the analysis. There was a very prolonged overidealization and overcathexis of the father image which Mahler (1966) has said occurs when there are "circumstances when the belief in magical omnipotence is not gradually replaced by secondary narcissism and autonomous ego development; instead, there is the acute threat of collapse of the feeling of omnipotence which has to be counteracted by overidealization and overcathexis of the father image" (p. 637). Mahler also refers to "a second instance of hypercathexis of the father image" which occurs "when sexualization, by way of primal scene observations or other traumatic overstimulation makes splitting of the father image necessary. In this case the sexual, hence 'bad', father image becomes massively repressed and the glorification of the split off, *asexual*, hence overidealized and 'good', father image is tenaciously maintained and defended" (ibid).

His concept of the perfect father weakened somewhat when Donald began to establish friendships with girls. With some difficulty, Donald said he had a new friend in school—a girl but not a girl friend. He was silent for a while and then blurted out that he could not come for his next few appointments for it would not be convenient for his father to drive him. After further silence, Donald flushed and admitted that his father had said no such thing but that he, that is, Donald, had "just thought it."

I commented that Donald was finding it hard to come now because he himself was worried about the changes going on in him, and he was not sure how his father or I would feel about these changes—his improvement in school, his having a friend who was a girl, and his greater freedom. I told Donald that he was not at ease with these changes in himself and really felt as though he should not enjoy life so much.

Donald picked up my mention of the girl and said: "I just knew you would make a big deal of that. She is not a girl friend. You Freudians always conjure up that nonsense." After another silence, he said: "You may be right. My father drove past me when I was talking to a girl. I don't know whether he saw me, but I felt very funny. I felt that way before, but I can't remember when." Later, he added: "This is not what I am trying to remember, but I felt funny the other day when I was hurrying my father because I thought I would be late for my appointment and my father said, 'You really want to get there, don't you?' "

Now Donald said that he had a "kookie" thought and although it did not make sense to him, he knew that I would feel it was important. "It was about the tantrums. I pictured myself hollering bad words near the wall and my mother got so upset. But my father was never home."

With some surprise, Donald now realized that his tantrums occurred only when his father worked at night and did not come home until well after Donald's bedtime. Donald added that on these nights his mother gave him dancing lessons in the basement and seemed warm and seductive, dancing very closely. If his father returned home early, his mother would turn off the music abruptly and send Donald to his room. Although Donald felt angry and strangely guilty, he did not have a tantrum. He interjected that this was the feeling he had been unable to remember when he told me of his father driving past him when he was speaking to a girl. He returned to the subject of his tantrums which always occurred when his father stayed out very late. It was obvious that they represented an orgastic, aggressive explosion and also served the purpose of alienating his mother, causing her to be so angry that she would stay away from him. Eventually, the tantrums kept his father at home.

I commented on the connection between the tantrums and Donald's excitement and guilt, summing up what Donald had told me: that although he could recall the pain and frustration which he experienced when his mother alternately wooed and rejected him, he was now aware that the anxiety was greater when his father worked late and his mother did not cast him off. Donald associated next to his plight with girls, telling me that since he expected rejection it was necessary to ward them off in advance. He said plaintively: "If you can't trust your mother, who can you trust?" He then made an unconscious slip: "Your mother can't trust you." Donald flushed and stammered and was extremely uneasy in response to this slip. He said that maybe he had to push his mother away since his father was not there to put Donald in his place, and, even if his father were there, he probably would not be effective.

After two years in analysis, Donald overidealized his father less and was more concerned about his father's passivity. Donald recalled having considered his father to be a "second Schweitzer." Now he wondered if, like Schweitzer, his father wanted him to be little, meek, and weak, for a book he had read criticized Schweitzer for his disinterest in improving the political status of the Africans and, instead, preferring them to be downtrodden.

Donald's size, which his mother had ridiculed, was also a component of his intrapsychic conflict with his father. Donald towered over both parents. His height and increasing strength contributed to a resurgence of childhood fantasies in which he exchanged places with his father. He would be big and his father little. To make father little was intolerable. His discomfort with largeness reinforced his need to be the innocent, unknowing, and suffering little boy.

Approximately six months later, a repetitive phenomenon appeared in the transference. Donald began each Monday session in identical fashion. He would slump in his chair, looking depressed and then proclaim: "I had a terrible weekend." However, his description of the weekend's events made it obvious that Donald was now embarking upon new and interesting adventures. He described pleasure in playing cards with his friends, accepting rides on a motorcycle, going to movies, and even attending a synagogue dance. I confronted Donald with this configuration, commenting that he was trying hard to convince me that he was miserable when he was, in fact, enjoying new experiences and having fun. Donald seemed quite surprised as he recognized: "That's what I tell my parents—that I had a terrible weekend. I guess I feel that you won't really like me or be interested in me if I say I have fun."

I recalled our previous conversation in which Donald had told me that he felt his parents were kind and tender when he was stupid, sick, or suffering but that, when he had a friend who was a girl, he was not sure that father or I liked that. He seemed to fear that everyone would be indifferent to him if he enjoyed himself. Donald associated to my comment by recalling that I seemed very indifferent to him early in his analysis when I did not appear overly sympathetic to his suffering. Often he felt that I just did not care what happened to him, in contrast to his father, who panicked when Donald was upset, and to his mother, who was affectionate when he was most disturbed.

Donald said that his father now hovered over him in a "very funny way." He seemed to ask him about his weekend plans as if he did not want Donald to go out at all. His father expressed disapproval and alarm if he felt that Donald would be too much on his own, or that he might do something wild or dangerous. Consequently, each Friday, Donald told his parents he had nothing to do and when they asked later what he had done, he merely said: "I had a terrible weekend." Donald went on to say that he really would not want me to hover over him or to "give him a Purple Heart for his suffering," but he continued to have the funny feeling that he would make me mad if he enjoyed himself.

I verbalized his ambivalence as it was expressed in the transference. Donald wished me to be very sympathetic when he was upset, yet he knew that it would not be helpful to him. He also expected me to disapprove of his weekend expeditions yet, at the same time, to foster them. Donald struggled with very real conflicts, for there was, indeed, disapproval with a concomitant withdrawal of both parents as he improved. A third source of conflict was his increased freedom and pleasure.

Donald began, at 17-1/2, to go out with girls, at first with little success, for his continuing defensive "toughness" and sarcasm made them unwilling to date him a second time. Soon Donald reported, with some embarrassment, that he was particularly interested in his boy friends' girls; at first he was aware that he was creating a triangle, and soon he was amazed to realize that he was jealous of both the girl and the boy. He derided each one of the dating pair to the other and recognized that he was thus trying to separate them. He suddenly remembered something which he had not "truly forgotten," but which he had neglected to tell me. It was that he had slept with one or the other parent from age 7 to 14. (His parents had never told me this.) The rationale for the sleeping arrangement had been that Donald's severe hay fever necessitated that he sleep in an air conditioned room! Winter and summer, Donald had slept in his parents' bedroom with one parent, while the other had been relegated to Donald's room. This practice had ceased the year before the start of his analysis. Donald had told his parents that they should buy an air conditioner for his room.

Soon after this disclosure, Donald confessed that for months he had been stalking his friends at night. He would slink around the neighborhood and, much like a peeping tom, peer through the windows of his friends' houses to see if a party were going on unbeknownst to him. Quite late, after the members of his crowd had gone their separate ways, he had a strong feeling that there was yet another party they had not told him about. In addition, he also revealed that he and his friends took great pleasure in breaking up parties, usually parties to which they had not been invited. They would create such a ruckus that the parents of the host or hostess would order everyone out. I commented to Donald that what he had just told me must be connected with the recent material about the sleeping arrangements of his family.

Donald now remembered that, as a child, he sometimes had awakened late at night to find the other twin bed empty. He recalled his fury and sense of having been betrayed. He then recalled that he had listened, his ear against the wall adjoining his parents' bedroom, for what he now understood had been primal scene sounds.

This sneaking and listening was reenacted in the transference when Donald began to phone me at two or three o'clock in the morning. If I answered, he would make a lame excuse for the call, usually questioning me about the time of his next appointment. If my husband answered, Donald would quietly hang up. When I confronted Donald with this behavior, Donald said he felt that when I answered, I really must be alone or asleep and I was certainly not betraying him; but when my husband answered, he felt that I had broken his trust in me. His affect was so reminiscent of his feeling of betrayal, when he had awakened alone as a child, that I told Donald his calling me late at night was similar to his curiosity and anger when he had found the twin bed empty. I added that he must have had a similar ''betrayal feeling'' when he fantasied about my sexual relationship with my husband. Donald denied that he had any such fantasies but now recalled once more, with glee, the parties that he and his friends had disrupted. He went on to say that he felt that any connection between breaking up parties in his neighborhood and calling me at night was very abstract. Since I might be inclined to believe this, he was denying it in advance. However, he very soon revealed that he had become quite uneasy with his English teacher after he had recognized her resemblance to me. He had begun to follow her around the campus (he was now in college) and tried to eat lunch where she did. After having seen her in a restaurant with a young man whom he identified as her fiance, Donald found himself furious, as though she had cheated him by not keeping a promise. He wondered if her fiance resembled my husband. This material was followed by a "still" dream which was in vivid color. (Previous analysis of his "still" dreams had clearly established that they were primal scene dreams where the accent on "still" served to deny movement.) Donald reported:

> We had an appointment and we were talking about something that was very pertinent and very shocking. I can't remember what. Maybe it had to do with why I'm having trouble reciting in English class. There was a snow storm after the appointment so I missed the next session. I went to my friend's house and I thought my father would take me to the appointment and he didn't and I had to take the bus and I was late. It was twelve-thirty P.M. and I didn't get to the appointment.

He interjected: "I've had the feeling my father is angry with me, like your husband." He went on:

> The next part was the still dream. You were angry at me and said: "You have to be punished. You have to find out something." Then I had to play being a doctor, but not as you. This is hard to explain—I had to catch someone in a restaurant. I can't remember their names but I knew them before I went to the restaurant. Before I went to the restaurant you had told me I was to fight two people, both me. One was in a suit and both had Mitch Miller beards; the other was heavier and quieter

but looked the same. The restaurant had cloths on the tables, not a place for kids. It was like one that you would go to.

Donald's associations led to heterosexual and homosexual fantasies. He brought up primal scene material through relating to the "still dreams," like still movies. As he had done before, he emphasized the absence of movement. Finally, he was able to recall that his previous insistence that a dream was "still" denied the more exciting movements. He associated to his father's not driving him to the appointment with the awareness of his father's growing hurt and anger as Donald needed him less. Now, Donald spent more time with his peers and performed better at school. Also, Donald thought he remembered that his father may have been angry when Donald interrupted him while he was in the next room.

Playing doctor brought up memories of mutual exploratory play with little girls. Donald recalled his horrified wonderment at seeing girls' genitals. The Mitch Miller beard referred to pubic hair, to his impression of father's large hairy genitals when Donald was little; then to his own sexual development which, so early in Donald's life, changed him from an innocent good boy into a hairy boy with large genitals. To the fighting, he associated his primal scene fantasies and wrestling with his father as a child. To my anger in the dream, he associated to the funny feelings he had when he and his father wrestled. It was a mixture of excitement and apprehension, but he could not fathom why I would order him to fight. He thought I might be angry about his curiosity and yet I ordered him to find things out. Donald could finally acknowledge having sexual curiosity about my marriage and wondering about my sexual life; he added that it must be "okay" to be curious because that was what analysis was all about.

After three years of treatment, the analysis had enabled Donald to work through his previous pathological certainty that his neighbors hated him and spied on him. The paranoid accusations had persisted but with less force. Donald continued to worry about his and my neighbors spying on him, although he gradually became less troubled. I reviewed the recent material about his wish to break up couples, his breaking up parties, his memories of listening at the wall adjoining his parents' bedroom, and his calling me late at night. Donald acknowledged his shame and guilt at listening as well as his fury when he felt betrayed. He seemed puzzled and said that he could understand everything except his accusations against the neighbors. He asked me, "Why the neighbors?" I did not answer and Donald, after a pause, went on to say: "They were always the enemy, I guess. She never liked them or trusted them, you know. She told me not to trust them. When I was little she told me never to take food from them, like they'd poison me. Like some nut put poison in trick or treat candy. She said that she would just know it happened." Then Donald added with a grin, "I guess they really were not listening, but if they were, I gave them something to listen to."

I pointed out to Donald that he had put the neighbors in the position of the excited, upset, and guilty child he had once been when he listened at the walls and did not quite know what was going on. Donald agreed and then said, "Boy, they must have thought there was a deluxe battle going on." I said: "As you thought sometimes when you listened." Donald flushed and then said with some embarrassment, "I just had a funny thought. Like maybe I saved you when I called late at night. Like maybe you were being hurt."

It was evident to Donald that his own excited listening against the wall had caused intolerable guilt and fury which he had to project onto his neighbors. In an exhibitionistic way, he enacted for them his erotic and sadistic fantasies of what transpired in the other bedroom. When the closeness to his mother became too stimulating, he shouted obscenities to ward her off.

By accusing his neighbors, Donald had been able to deny and

project onto them his own dirty curiosity. He turned passive into active when he became the participant rather than the audience. In his furious tantrums, not only did he reenact primal scenes with his mother, but he expressed marked sadism toward her, for he well knew her vulnerability in respect to her enormous fear of her neighbors' criticism. And finally, there were components of identification with his mother's paranoia.

Sometime later, through word usage and grammar, Donald revealed a need to ward me off when he felt too stimulated in the analytic hours. Again, there was identification with his mother, although not with her psychotic projections. A well-read boy, Donald could express himself with elegance, but there were times when he spoke like a slum child, using such expressions as: "He done it real good." When I commented on this, Donald at first denied that either such extreme of usage ever occurred. Later, he associated to his mother's idiomatic expressions; not having completed high school she spoke quite ungrammatically. When Donald spoke or wrote well, and especially if he criticized his mother, she would say sarcastically: "This is what you are learning at school—to know more than your mother. Soon you'll be too good for me." I pointed out that Donald used poor grammar to convince his mother and himself that he had not developed beyond her; I also recalled that he had told me of having used vile language to ward her off when they were too close at night. Donald answered that, although he no longer had temper tantrums, he had to shout obscenely, even now, to get his mother out of his bedroom. She came to his room in a flimsy nightgown for the purpose of adjusting the window ventilators. Donald insisted that he had to swear at her in order "to get her angry enough" to leave. I told Donald that it seemed, then, that his use of poor grammar here in the office must have somewhat the same purpose as it did at home. I added that when we spoke of his sexual feelings, Donald reacted at times as though I were encouraging him to be bad or dirty. Donald said that he could not accept this. He immediately associated to a friend's ribald comments when he had heard that Donald was seeing a woman psychiatrist. Donald said that what his friend had described was too bad to tell me but sometimes his friend teased him by suggesting that a woman psychiatrist would be seductive with him. Eventually, Donald realized that he employed the low-class speech in the office to tell me that both he and I were low-class and to "cool" things when he had upsetting sexual fantasies about me.

Donald's interest in schoolwork now expanded greatly. A sophomore in college, he evidenced for the first time an intense interest in history. That this subject inevitably brought conflicts to the fore was revealed by Donald's complaints that reading history caused him to have severe headaches. In pursuing this, I asked Donald what aspect of history he found especially interesting. Donald complained at first of my having to know "every last thing he was interested in." He seemed unusually resistive to discussing what bothered him so much, whereupon I said that analysis and history were rather alike, for they both dealt with what had happened in the past and how the past affected the present. Donald laughed apprehensively and said: "So you are saying that analysts are curious too." I agreed and added that Donald, however, was telling me that his curiosity stirred up conflicts since he developed such bad headaches. He told me he was fascinated by books on the Italian-Ethiopian War and on ancient Egyptian practices. The headaches occurred after he had read of the Ethiopians' punishment of the captured Italians by castration, and the disclosure of father-daughter or brother-sister marriages among the Egyptian royalty. The headaches were dissipated after he had disclosed that the reading resulted in exciting and frightening fantasies in which castration was the punishment both for his aggression and his incestuous thoughts which were stirred up when he read of the marriage practices of the Egyptian royalty.

A new phase in the analysis was introduced when Donald told me how upset he became when he read about the ancient Grecian gymnasia and the freedom of men at that time to love each other. Donald expressed disgust and distress about the nudity of the men and said that he felt it was awful that a civilization should have existed which had accepted male homosexuality and even promoted it. However, it was soon apparent that Donald was acting out homosexual fantasies. He wandered around the center of the city late at night, dressed in tight dungarees and sneakers, the costume of the male homosexual. At first, he complained that homosexuals made verbal overtures to him; soon he realized that he was asking for such episodes to happen. With considerable anxiety, he explained that he was having masturbation fantasies that must mean he was a "fag." He was on the bottom while a big man lay atop him, still. Our previous analysis of still dreams enabled Donald to know that "motionless" meant just the opposite. He associated to having slept, in his early years, with his father who had comforted him and had lain close to him, often sleeping nude. Donald recalled two opposing reactions to having seen his father's genitals. He had been overwhelmed by their size and had felt inadequate since his own penis was so much smaller. On the other hand, he had felt happy that his father had a penis and did not have deformed genitals as did his mother. With great discomfort, Donald recalled the desire to be penetrated by his father's penis, and his childhood wish to touch it. Donald then said that only a woman could touch anything in his family. The dreams and fantasies slowly changed to scenes in which Donald was the aggressor while another, unrecognized male, was the receptive "woman with a vagina."

At this time, Donald reported that he refused to sit on the living room floor but sat on the sofa instead. His father followed his lead and his mother "backed down." Donald was proud of his masculine role but expressed guilt at having put father down. He felt his father was too weak to be the man with mother, and that he was unable to keep Donald from overstepping oedipal boundaries. With guilt, Donald began to acknowledge that sometimes he had requested the dancing lessons. He recalled his sexual excitement and again recognized his tantrums as an enactment of the primal scene. He could finally (after three and a half years in analysis) discuss what he called his mother's "nutty beliefs." He was saddened that she continued to say her neighbors spied on her and snubbed her and he recognized that her problems were instrumental in creating the difference between the neighbors and herself. He recalled that she had been overly critical of everyone, including himself. He returned to the fear that no one would love him since he was so ugly. His continuing fear of homosexuality, and his growing awareness of his erotic feelings toward his mother, were apparent in a letter Donald sent me while I was on my summer vacation:

Dear Dr. Kramer:
I hope that you are enjoying your vacation. I hate to bother you with a problem but it has become serious. I am now working for ———— Service. My job is to deliver packages to stores with a driver from a tractor trailer. This man, a Negro, has me disturbed and it may cost me my job. He is a married man and he goes out with other women. Not only that, but he describes his sexual experiences with me and asks me to describe mine to him. I am starting to use his filthy language around the house and talk rough around girls because I feel that if he can pick up girls by talking like this maybe I could. I think that I am trying to prove that to hang around this type of person will make me dirty too. It hinders my relationship with him and makes me tense at work. I wonder how friendly I can become with him since I must work all day with him. I feel somewhat guilty that I envy him somehow.
At home I have noticed that sometimes I become affectionate with mom without any response from her. This gets me angry at her. I want a date with a girl more than ever now. Work is making me more girl conscious.

I had a dream that a big, intelligent giant exchanged my brain for his. It must have been my father, although I can't understand it. It is very obvious that I am now seeking feminine affection and treat mom like I would like to treat a girl.

I guess that's all that has come up in the last few days. I would like your advice concerning the Negro driver, as my attitude concerning him is puzzling.

Maybe you could write me a letter or suggest some other way of getting in touch with you, such as your phone number, if you have one at your home. I would appreciate some advice greatly.

Yours truly,
Donald

I called Donald from my vacation home and found that a phone conversation was sufficient to alleviate a mounting panic. The letter was dealt with extensively after my vacation. Donald blamed me for freeing him to work with the Negro who excited him sexually, stirred up homosexual and heterosexual fantasies, and evoked his desire to emulate him. The driver's openness about his sexual escapades and Donald's wish to be like him were threatening to Donald, who accused me of abandoning him while I was having a good time over the summer.

Donald was pleased that the driver, by questioning him about his sexual exploits, had implied that he was capable of attracting girls and having intercourse. He was, however, humiliated by the fact that he was still a virgin. In the transference, Donald realized that he was angry with me for having deserted him when I was away with my husband. He said angrily: "I know you want me to say I thought about you and your husband on a vacation together." He added sarcastically, "No, I guess I should think that you went to a psychiatric meeting and left your husband home." I said, "Like when you hoped your parents were apart at night?" Donald seemed embarrassed and said: "To make sure, I called you once at night and no one answered for a long time. I thought that maybe your husband would answer but it was your answering service, so I knew you were away together.'' He then added that this telephone incident had resulted in fantasies of my having a wild fling with my husband who (together with his father and the driver) was the man with whom Donald had exchanged his brain in the dream. After a while, Donald said that possibly his worrisome letter was like the old pronouncement ''I had an awful weekend,'' for he really had enjoyed the summer more than any other previous one. Now Donald could discuss heterosexual masturbatory fantasies involving classmates and it was obvious that there was a spurt in his development.

Donald was increasingly active with girl friends and dated each week. He no longer used the ''I had a terrible weekend'' approach, but reported his dating experiences honestly. He seemed to be able to interest girls and to carry a relationship beyond the initial stages. Nonetheless, he experienced mounting anxiety when he knew the girl well enough to kiss her good night or to fondle her. When he first attempted to touch his date's genitals and she responded by touching his clothed penis, Donald experienced a severe panic and took her home immediately. He did not report this to me at the time, but showed himself to be increasingly upset in the transference.

Second Paranoid Phase

Donald had been in analysis approximately four and a half years when he manifested a second episode of regression. He revealed somatic delusions as he accused me of knowing, but of refusing to admit to him, that I saw his lips and nose become markedly swollen and then return to normal size. The overt disclosure of the delusions was triggered by my questioning Donald about his need to wear sunglasses in the office. Although he responded to my first inquiries with an offhand ''I just like to wear them,'' Donald realized by now that this behavior contained an analytic meaning. He finally blurted out that they were to keep people from knowing what he was thinking. He associated to his fear of his gentile uncle at whose undressed wife Donald had peeped when he was a young child. Donald thought that my husband must be gentile and he assumed that he must be the elderly handyman working on the grounds. He added also that my husband must stay at home to keep an eye on things in case any of my patients became unruly and "fresh." He had fantasies of being chased by his virile uncle whose wife had ten children, a fact which Donald regarded as a testimony to his uncle's masculinity. Donald told me that he had hated being Jewish, for Jews were weak and impotent, not sexually potent and strong like his uncle.

Donald now reported that he was exceedingly uncomfortable when asked to recite in school for he was sure that he would make an "ass" of himself and everyone would know that he was a "jerk off." This was followed by the emergence of paranoid-like material which was now confined to the analysis. Donald told me that he thought I was smiling sarcastically as if I knew something about him and were sneering at him. He was accusatory and angry with me and at the same time beseeched me not to be critical of him. Although his mother's sneering expressions and constant use of sarcasm had come up in the analysis repeatedly, Donald was not able to make use of our past work to understand his thought regarding me as a transference manifestation. He accused me, over and over again, of laughing at him. When I told him that the only way in which he would be able to understand this thought would be by associating to it, Donald said that he knew I knew all his secrets and that I must be keeping from him the fact that I could see his nose and lips become swollen and unswollen. He insisted that I knew what he meant for he could see me watching his face and he knew that I was keeping my knowledge from him.

He then recalled that his mother had often told him that she knew his pimples were from bad thoughts and bad feelings and that she could tell what he had been up to by looking at his face. I pointed out that Donald seemed to feel that I, too, could look at his face and know what was going on in his mind. He was sure that I knew what he was up to and even what his genitals were experiencing. Donald said that he had assumed all along that sometimes I might read his mind, although he knew I could not. Yet when I made interpretations to him that clarified things he had not known, he thought that I must have a magical touch. This was not really unlike what his mother had indicated that she had when she had said she knew when he was lying because she could read it all over his face.

Donald next said that in early adolescence, after he had masturbated into his underpants, his mother had told him not to blow his nose or to spit into his clothing. Donald knew that his mother knew what he was doing. He acknowledged that a kind of unspoken pact kept each of them from speaking openly of his masturbation.

For some six months, Donald continued his unshaken belief that I must be able to see the changes in his nose and lips. Only after I had told Donald that he could be transferring to me a real experience from his childhood, did he associate to the fact that his mother had bathed him until he was past 12 years old, scrubbing his entire body to prevent him from getting acne. Donald had reached puberty at 9-1/2 and he found these baths to be exquisitely painful and threatening as well as exciting. He was ashamed that he enjoyed his mother's touch on his genitals, yet he was angry because, by her casual touching, she behaved as though he did not have anything there. The collusion of his mother with Donald in denying the source of the wetness of the underpants, and in the upward displacement of his badness to his acne-covered face, reinforced an almost *folie à deux* expectation that certain women, his mother and I, both dangerously seductive women, had magical powers. We could tell what Donald was thinking and what his genitals experienced. After I had interpreted this fantasy, Donald could acknowledge his mingled pleasure and tension when he talked of sexual matters with me. He continued to speak of his certainty that I saw the changing size of his lips and nose.

I commented that Donald feared that speaking of sexual material might cause him to have an erection here, reminding him of the worrisome and exciting baths. He agreed, and then said: "She touched my penis and ignored my erection, like it was nothing, like it was too little to acknowledge." I pointed out that Donald felt that women were seductive and cruel at the same time, that they both excited and demeaned him. He was not only angry at women, he was also angry at himself for liking and tolerating the baths with mother and the stimulating talks with me. To this, Donald said: "She knew and she sneered at me. She thought I was dirty and made me go to the acne doctor before I had even begun to develop. She told me in advance that I'd be dirty." Here, I referred to the previous material concerning his masturbating in his underpants, and Donald said, "Of course, I had to masturbate after I got excited. So I would get out of the bath and I never felt clean because I had dirty feelings and I always felt dirtier after I mastur-bated."

Donald's delusions that I could see his nose and lips undergo tumescence and detumescence slowly disappeared as he continued to discuss memories of actual stimulation by his overtly prim and proper mother. In the transference, he experienced the fears and expectations that I would stimulate him by toying with his mind as his mother had done with his body. Then I would sneeringly humiliate him by treating him as though he were only that dirty little boy, of no sexual consequence whatsoever. I referred to his fantasies that my husband stayed around to keep an eye on things, saying that Donald might have been reassured if this were true. Donald agreed on two scores: first, this would have meant that I considered Donald a sexual adult who could do something; and second, Donald would have known that he could not get away with being fresh although, he assured me, he would not have tried anything.

There followed a resurgence of earlier material about his mother's disdain of him as the pimply, dirty boy who was worth nothing, a castrate. He was angry again because his father had not protected him from the sarcastic, sneering mother. Finally, Donald said: "He wasn't the man to handle her." His awareness that he was stronger than his father briefly stirred homosexual fantasies with Donald in the role of aggressor. Heterosexual fantasies and age appropriate heterosexual play followed. He finally divested me of my magical powers and no longer felt that I was secretly hiding things from him.

Now, Donald was self-critical as he dealt with his wish that I would stimulate him and with his awareness of the exhibitionism implicit in his imploring me to look at him. The strictness of his superego was not reduced until the later analysis of his identification with the self-punishing and self-denying attributes of his father.

Terminal Phase

In spite of our previous work, Donald repeated at times that he found it hard to believe that I could accept him "in his dirtiness" and that I was not repelled by his acne. I talked to Donald about the rigorous treatment for the acne; and of his disappointment that such extremes of self-denial had brought no improvement in his skin, for Donald had adhered to an unbelievably limited diet. Now, past 20, Donald was tempted to break the diet. He began to drink whole milk and to eat butter for the first time since he was 8-1/2. Since we had talked of the strictness of the diet in the analysis, Donald felt, of course, that I was encouraging him to cheat. Donald's anger at his mother for enforcing his diet was expressed almost daily, but his dilemma about eating adequately was not resolved for many months. It was through analysis of the eating practices in the family that Donald finally began to see his parents more objectively and to separate from their pathology.

Donald complained that I encouraged him to break his diet. In actuality, I did find it difficult to avoid going counter to the extremely rigid dietary limitations imposed upon him, first by the dermatologist and then by his mother. However, I felt that Donald had to analyze his need to conform to every nuance of the diet as would few boys at his age. His obvious fear of incurring the wrath of his mother, and of the maternal components of his superego, was rather easily handled, as was his expectation that his skin would worsen if he defied the dermatologist.

However, the glory he experienced in self-deprivation, in identification with his father, complicated this food problem. It was brought into the analysis when, in extreme opposition to his previous habit of wearing sun glasses everywhere, Donald began wearing them not at all, not even in the brightest sunlight. During the summer, Donald would arrive blinking and uncomfortable, but he would say then that he felt it was "sissy" to wear sun glasses. Along the same vein, Donald denied himself the comfort and protection of a raincoat or umbrella in a severe downpour. After I had pointed out the number of ways in which he called attention to his self-neglect, Donald told me that his father never used sun glasses, umbrella, or raincoat, for to use these was unmanly.

Donald was defensive when he told me of his father's beliefs. When I pointed to his defensiveness, he said that he thought I might encourage him to take the easy way out—to wear sun glasses and to eat differently. He went on to describe his father as a stoic who complained of nothing, not even his diet. Donald revealed that his mother had imposed upon his father a low cholesterol diet lest someday he develop high cholesterol, have a heart attack, and die. Donald's and his father's diets were quite similar, as completely free of fats as possible (Donald, who was over six feet tall, weighed one hundred and thirty-five pounds.) The food father and son ate was broiled or boiled, lacking fats and seasoning. Donald realized that he was always hungry and always angry. He blamed the analysis for making him aware of both his hunger and his anger and said that I did not tell him how to solve the eating problem, only to be aware of it.

Donald began to block during his hours, to be occasionally

silent, and to forget what was on his mind. When I commented that he seemed, at the same time, both to want and not to want to tell me something, he confessed to having eaten hamburgers and french fried potatoes for the first time in his life. He was contrite and yet very elated, especially when his acne improved. Soon afterward, to his horror and delight, when he and his friends were in a diner, he spotted his father eating a cheeseburger. Donald did not confront his father with this encounter, but he discussed it in the analysis. It was very painful for him to realize that his father's meekness, and his refusal or inability to stand up to his mother, had given Donald a distorted concept of what was manly. Donald knew that his father felt he should not protect himself against harsh weather and associated to the fact that he protected neither himself nor Donald when he acquiesced to the diets, or to sitting on the living room floor. Donald's growing awareness of his father's weakness left him feeling unprotected against his mother's need to control every facet of his life. He eventually realized that he was stronger than his father and that women were witches only when men allowed them to be. At this point, Donald realized that he had not been manipulated by his mother's needs alone, but much of their interaction had been motivated by his own needs to be stimulated, punished, and controlled.

Donald spent a long time in typical adolescent disillusionment with his parents, with depression, as he separated from these ambivalently cathected primary love objects. As he divested his mother of the superstrength, superrightness, and remnants of magical omnipotence which he had attributed to her, he felt alone, vulnerable, and incapable of making independent judgments.

It is significant that although he seemed to share only his mother's distorted, psychotic thinking in the early stages of analysis, in the later stages it became clear that he clung tenaciously to elements of his father's thinking that were quite bizarre.

Detachment from his father was slower and more tortuous than from his mother. One may speculate that he was able to see me as a substitute as he withdrew from the painful, humiliating, infantilizing sadomasochistic relationship with his mother. Although many adolescent boys decathect their fathers quite slowly, the slowness of the process was exaggerated in this case because of the multiple parental functions which Donald's father supplied for him. Further, Mr. Y's pathology was relatively subtle and innocuous, even noble in Donald's eyes. This was in contrast to Mrs. Y's obvious psychosis and her alternations of seduction and humiliation. Donald had a strong need to cling to the nurturing provided by his father whom he hero-worshipped. Their relationship was threatened both internally and externally by Donald's painful awareness of his father's need to keep him dependent, and by the slow admission to himself that his father distorted reality in no small degree.

A major obstacle was Donald's discomfort in acknowledging his father's passivity, for this connoted a passive feminine identity in both his father and himself. When Donald recognized that he was the more manly of the two, danger of oedipal victory was revived. This danger was attenuated by the fact that Donald was able to make a nonincestuous object choice as he dated regularly and successfully with the young woman whom he later married.

Reality pressures added to the problems of detachment from his father. In contrast to his mother, who, perhaps not too surprisingly, took pride in her son's greater effectiveness, especially when he was the first cousin to become engaged, his father withdrew from Donald into a hurt, sullen detachment. It seemed as though Mr. Y suffered, for the second time, the disappointment of the loss of his father-companion and the angry depression he had experienced when his own father had remarried.

SUMMARY

I have described in detail two episodes of severe ego regression in the course of a long analysis of an adolescent boy. In each episode there was a partial impairment of reality testing and a use of pathological defenses. The second incident revealed somatic delusions, with difficulty in differentiating self and object.

The ubiquitousness of phase-specific regression as a normal part of adolescence, without which the developmental tasks of this phase of life cannot be accomplished, have been well described by A. Freud (1958), Geleerd (1957, 1961), Spiegel (1951, 1958), and Blos (1967). Pathological regression during adolescence is discussed in vignettes of cases by Spiegel (1958), Laufer (1968), and Blos (1967). In formulating the genesis of severe ego regression, the authors find that their cases have in common a history of severe pre-oedipal traumata, very often with "excessive and repeated premature genital arousal" (Harley, 1970, p. 110).

Laufer describes a crucial conflict in some adolescents over whether the now mature body belongs to them or to their mothers who first cared for it. He believes that the regressive fantasies and memories of pre-oedipal experiences were finally brought to light in the transference phenomenon. This was especially so in the second regressive episode in Donald's analysis, where he experienced considerable doubt as to the "ownership of his body."

I wish to repeat here the fact that the ego regression was partial. Even before the regressive episodes came into the analysis, Donald was able to perform better in school, to make new friends, to start the slow process which finally enabled him to become increasingly independent of early object ties, and to tolerate those temporary increases of anxiety or anger stirred by the analytic process. Throughout the analysis, he was able to sustain a good therapeutic relationship. Identification with me occurred, permitting the observing part of Donald's ego to ally itself with that of the analyst. The evidence of the usable therapeutic relationship, as well as manifestations of improved ego functioning as the analysis proceeded, enabled me to be confident that analysis was the treatment of choice.

I feel that I must include mention here that a transference

neurosis existed among the multiplicity of relationships to me that developed in the course of Donald's analysis. I agree with Scharfman (1971), who wonders at the absence of reported cases of transference neurosis in adolescents. Scharfman says: "The clinical transference picture can very often be obscured by the fact that the phase-specific libidinal push and the defense attempts to deal with it involve the analyst in additional roles . . . the analyst may be not only transference object, or object of displacement, he may also be 'new' object."

An important collection of case vignettes presented to the Kris Study Group, and reported by Joseph (1965), provide an excellent source of material concerning severe ego regression during psychoanalysis of patients who were chronologically adults. The anemneses reveal a failure of normal adolescence in all of the cases cited; these patients had remained extremely immature. Their analytic material included regressive fantasies which made obvious the fact that they could not distinguish inner from outer thoughts and feelings. All had episodes of poor reality testing. Some had somatic delusions that derived from early problems of body image. There were excesses of scoptophilia and exhibitionism, and a number of these patients found it difficult to distinguish self and object. The analyses produced evidence of repeated excessive overstimulation, dating back to the pre-oedipal period.

Similarities between the regression in the Kris Study Group cases and that evidenced by Donald are striking. We expect phase-specific regression in adolescents. Should we be surprised to encounter severe regressive phenomena in analysis of adolescents? I have been concerned with the attitude of child analysts who feel that adolescents cannot or should not be analyzed. Possibly the realization that severe regression does not mitigate against successful analysis may help to modify this attitude.

The Kris Study Group, referring to their adult patients, suggest that ego regression may be encountered in patients who range from healthy to those who demonstrate severe pathology. Severe ego regression may be seen in those whose pathology ranges from severe neuroses through borderline states to mild psychoses. They conclude that a longer than average analysis will be necessary. And they feel that the regressive phenomena must be analyzed like any other analytic material.

In Donald's case, one might have been cautious in attempting psychoanalysis in view of the severe parental pathology, the history of early and repeated traumata, and the danger of serious regression. Are we too pessimistic when we establish criteria for analyzability of adolescents? I hope that the variety of adolescent analyses described in this book may enable us to reconsider these stipulations and encourage us to analyze some adolescents who do not fit within the category of the "normal neurotic," and whose parents may not impress us most favorably.

BIBLIOGRAPHY

Blos, Peter. 1967. The second individuation process of adolescence. *Psychoanalytic Study of the Child* 22:162-86.

Freud, Anna. 1958. Adolescence. *Psychoanalytic Study of the Child* 13:225-78.

Geleerd, Elisabeth R. 1957. Some aspects of psychoanalytic technique in adolescence. *Psychoanalytic Study of the Child* 13:279-95.

———. 1961. Some aspects of ego vicissitudes in adolescence. *Journal of the American Psychoanalytic Association* 9:394-405.

Harley, Marjorie. 1970. On some problems of technique in the analysis of early adolescents. *Psychoanalytic Study of the Child* 25:99-121.

Joseph, Edward D., ed. 1965. Regressive ego phenomena in psychoanalysis. In *Monograph 1*, Monograph Series of the Kris Study Group of the New York Psychoanalytic Institute, pp. 68-103. New York: International Universities Press.

Laufer, Moses. 1968. The body image, the function of masturbation, and adolescence: Problems of the ownership of the body. *Psychoanalytic Study of the Child*, 23:114-37.

Mahler, Margaret S. 1942. Pseudo-imbecility: A magic cap of invisibility. *Psychoanalytic Quarterly* 11:149-64.

———. 1966. Discussion of "Problems of overidealization of the analyst and analysis." Presented at the New York Psychoanalytic Society, October 11, 1966. Abstracted in *Psychoanalytic Quarterly* 36:637.

Scharfman, M.A. 1971. Transference phenomena in adolescent analysis. In *The Unconscious Today*, ed. Mark Kanzer. New York: International Universities Press.

Spiegel, Leo A. 1951. A review of contributions to a psychoanalytic theory of adolescence: Individual aspects. *Psychoanalytic Study of the Child*, 6:375-93.

———. 1958. Comments on the psychoanalytic psychology of adolescence. *Psychoanalytic Study of the Child* 13:296-308.

Sprince, Marjorie P. 1967. The psychoanalytic handling of pseudo-stupidity and grossly abnormal behavior in a highly intelligent boy. In *The child analyst at work*, ed. Elisabeth Geleerd. New York: International Universities Press.

The Analysis of a
15-1/2-Year-Old Girl
with Suicidal Tendencies

Paulina F. Kernberg, M.D.   *Topeka*

INTRODUCTION

The analysis of an adolescent brings with it numerous problems of diagnosis and technique. The treatment described herein was no exception. However, psychoanalytic treatment of adolescents may be rewarding. According to Marjorie Harley (1965), during this period of life, we have material accessible which is the process of reorganization or attempts of reorganization. Further, the secondary or tertiary complications of the patient's neurosis through the choice of marital partners, children, and professional vocation are yet in the future, leaving at the patient's disposal the greatest range of freedom from neurotically determined decisions.

In this clinical presentation, I shall describe first the findings available to the analyst from the patient's initial consultation which led to the patient's referral for psychoanalytic treatment. I will then present selected vignettes from the treatment process, which will illustrate the theme of the patient's suicidal tendencies as it unfolded in the course of three years of treatment and five hundred and seventy hours. I have specifically selected the patient's suicidal tendencies because suicidal tendencies epitomize acting-

I am indebted to Dr. Gertrude Ticho for her valuable suggestions in my work with this patient.

out proclivities of adolescents and because an examination in depth of one case may complement the various studies on suicide in adolescents (Barter, 1959); Balser, 1968; Gould, 1965; Seiden, 1969; Teicher, 1966) which describe epidemiological, social and psychological factors. These authors have pointed out the following factors as particularly relevant in suicide problems in adolescents: first, the risk of suicide is greater in those adolescents who do not have an active social life and in those who live in a chaotic environment. In addition, there is increased risk if a person close to the child has died during the phallic and pubertal periods against a background of strong stimulation of the child's attachment to one of the parents. Various dynamic factors seem to play a role; the wish to gain support and strength through joining the powerful lost loved object; death as retaliation for abandonment; manipulation and blackmail to obtain love and attention and to punish a significant person; atonement for one's sins by dying; self-murder. Balser and Masterson (1959) add that depression is not an important factor in suicidal attempts during adolescence. Indeed, they have observed schizophrenic symptomatology more frequently than depressive symptomatology in adolescents.

I was surprised to find that practically all these dynamics, described in the literature in a wide variety of adolescent cases, could be found in this single case, in addition to still others. I believe this finding was possible because the analysis permitted the exploration of the various layers of the suicidal tendencies at different stages of regression within the transference neurosis.

Another finding which the clinical material illustrates is the changing form of the suicidal fantasy according to the degree of resolution of the patient's conflicts around her sexual identity.[1]

THE CASE

Alicia was a 15-1/2-year-old girl when she was first referred to a psychiatrist because her parents had been sufficiently alarmed by her suicidal threats to request psychiatric help. She had put her sister's jumping rope around her neck on several occasions, though this gesture seemed to her mother to lack real conviction. Two months prior to her initial consultation with a psychiatrist, she had become increasingly upset following the death of a close female relative who had died of cancer.

Alicia had become very antagonistic toward her parents; she felt she was not worth the money her parents spent on her. She even resented the food she was eating because "in Asia people have nothing to eat." She complained of being unloved and rejected by her parents, while at the same time feeling that her parents tried to run her life. She also complained of being rejected by her younger siblings. Of all her siblings, she felt closest to her brother Carlos, two years younger than herself.

Alicia came from a closely knit Spanish immigrant family. The closely knit interaction within the family was illustrated by the fact that the children had shared beds and bathroom until their teens, and by the blurring of generations as described by Theodore Lidz (1968).

Alicia's father, a pharmacologist in his forties, was extremely involved in his profession. He seemed to function best in emotionally neutral situations. At home he was either aloof or prone to outbursts of anger. Her mother was a constricted person who suffered from severe obesity and conversion symptoms such as numbness in her hands, and headaches. For many years, the mother would not leave her children with a babysitter. In fact, she seemed unable to talk about her children as separate individuals.

The mother's strong identification with Alicia could be illustrated by the way she described "how Alicia had asthma and was also so sensitive and was easily hurt, exactly like me." This same aspect of their relationship was illustrated by a fall that Alicia had sustained as a young girl. She had fallen down from a tree. The mother had come to her rescue and had started to cry. Alicia wondered why her mother was crying when, after all, it was she, Alicia, who was in pain.

The patient was the first child, born several years after the parents' marriage. Mother felt quite disappointed about having a girl, but tried not to show it (as her own mother had done with her). Labor was prolonged. Forceps had to be used, causing diffuse bruises and skin abrasions on Alicia's lips and face. As a result, the patient still had a hardly perceptible linear scar on her lower lip. Her lips were so affected that she had trouble nursing for a few days. Her birth weight was normal at full term. She was precocious in her developmental landmarks. Toilet training began at seven months and by sixteen months Alicia asked to be placed on the toilet seat. She was completely dry both day and night by eighteen months.

Alicia lived a rather isolated life, divided between school and home. Her relationship with her immediate younger brother was quite close. During high schools years, they spent most afternoons together doing their homework, with much teasing and bantering between them and a good bit of physical contact.

The first two and a half years of Alicia's life were spent uneventfully in a rather quiet and stable home atmosphere. One of her favorite memories was that of having welcomed her father upon his return from a trip, and she recalled how she had worn a blue dress and her favorite red shoes for that occasion. As the other siblings came along, her relationship with her parents became more strained. Her father's increasing involvement in his business made him less available to his family. Her mother felt lonely and became upset. Concomitantly, Alicia started to have temper tantrums which, during her preschool years, lasted at times for as long as two hours. These temper tantrums continued up to the time of the psychiatric examination in the form of temper outbursts which made her parents overly cautious in their interaction with her. By threatening, in her parents' presence, to put a jumping rope around her neck, Alicia was successful in forcing them to cease their arguments and quarrels.

In kindergarten, it became apparent that it was extremely difficult for Alicia to adjust to any new environment. She manifested this pattern throughout her school years, when changing from one school to another, and when the family moved to a new neighborhood.

Later, in elementary school, her learning was impaired to the extent that in spite of being considered a bright girl she averaged only C's in the first three grades. After that, she became an A and B student. By the time she ended junior high school, at age 13, she was considered a "loner." She complained about boys in school who teased her and used profane language against her, making her parents think that this was the reason for her troubles. During this period, some schoolmates made comments to her about the scar on her lips. According to the patient, this was the first time that she had realized she had such a scar. At this point, her mother had described for her rather vividly how she had been "a mess" when she was born, referring to the effects of the forceps.

Menarche occurred at age 13. Alicia was afraid of her periods and felt quite embarrassed not only by her menstruation, but also by the idea of sexual intercourse, which she thought was all right for animals, but not for humans. According to her parents, she had become aware of the sexual differences between her brother and herself as soon as her brother had been born. She planned never to get married or to have children.

Because of her food allergies, hay fever, and asthma, she had required allergy shots for several years.

Alicia's appearance was, in itself, a language of its own. Moderately obese, her hair and dress style reminded the interviewer of a little girl coming out of an orphanage. She moved around as if she did not deserve the space she occupied. This extreme of humbleness and humility had the secondary effect of especially attracting the attention of the examiner. Her appearance paralleled the appearance of her mother, whose obesity, unstylish and unbecoming dress disguised her more pleasant looks.

Alicia's initial consultation indicated that she was intelligent. She was able to establish good contact with me. She showed a certain ability to look at things in her life from different points of view. For example, she could admit that something within herself prevented her from remembering sexual information. She used fantasy and humor quite readily. Affect seemed to be accessible to her, and she presented a variety of moods such as sadness, humor, teasing, despair, embitterment, and self-depreciatory feelings. Aggression seemed to be strongly warded off by reversal, reaction formations and by masochistic features as illustrated by her accounts of numerous minor accidents which she described as amusing anecdotes. There was a hidden pleasure and satisfaction on being teased by others and in presenting herself as an utterly unattractive and deprived girl.

Alicia's physical symptoms and allergies provided the secondary gain of having her father around, because he was always there only when "you are sick." These symptoms also served as rationalizations of her inhibitions, especially in her social life. Thus, supposedly she could not date because she could not go out of the house lest she would have an asthmatic attack. Although she was withdrawn socially, in fantasy she was quite invested in other people. She was keenly aware of the examiner's person.

Alicia was also aware that she had problems, that she "just could not outgrow her problems" by herself like "the majority of teenagers would." The conviction of this statement was put to test by the fact that four months elapsed before I could start her psychoanalytic treatment. By that time, she was feeling in a much better mood. She had a volunteer job and felt that she was being useful and helpful. Yet, she persisted in her intent of initiating her treatment. When her schedule of five weekly sessions was discussed, she was quite cooperative in spite of some realistic difficulties. She revealed her conflicts about being a patient by stating that she would like to be a psychiatrist to resolve her own problems.

It was felt that Alicia's superior intelligence, verbal ability, potential accessibility to affect, awareness of discomfort, wish for help, a certain sense of humor, and sublimatory capacities such as artistic activities and organization of capacities were all indications that she possessed the necessary ego capacities for psychoanalysis. It was also felt that psychoanalysis was the treatment of choice to prevent her further deterioration and to avoid her further withdrawal into fantasy, social isolation and an intensification of her suicidal trend.

Both parents had had psychotherapeutic treatment which had proved to be helpful to them. This provided a good basis for their conscious cooperation and acceptance of the patient's analysis. The parents terminated their own casework treatment one year before Alicia's termination of her treatment.[2]

I will now present a series of vignettes of selected sessions in chronological order so as to highlight the meaning and technical handling of Alicia's suicidal threats throughout her analysis and up to the point of termination. Theoretical considerations will be included in my later discussion.

Alicia did not use the couch initially. Instead, she spontaneously sat with her face turned away from the analyst. She stated quite explicitly that if she became too comfortable, as she might become by using the couch, she might be "carried away and talk too much." After almost a year, when she had acquired more insight into the way in which she projected her aggression (she had been afraid of being "stabbed in the back" were she to use the couch), she made the decision to lie on the couch.

CLINICAL MATERIAL

The patient's suicidal tendencies (I include here both suicidal threats and suicidal attempts) represented a complex fantasy formation.

Already in the third hour, Alicia brought up the theme of death. Smiling rather sadly, she said that sometimes she had thought nobody really cared for her. Perhaps she would kill herself, and the only reason she had not killed herself was because of her pets. Her parents, she went on, kept saying that they loved her, but they had to; they were responsible for her. In school, she was just a number that handed in reports. When I asked whether she felt I could not care for her and would also see her as a number, she smiled sadly and said that she had thought about putting a rope around her neck, or picking up a gun, or using a knife but she did not know whether she would actually have the courage to kill herself. She liked the Catholic idea of death; when children die, they die because God wants them back.

At the beginning of the third week of her analysis, Alicia commented that she had had some "really strange" dreams the previous night. She had dreamed that she had been bitten on her arm by a snake and had gone to the emergency room of a general hospital where they did not have antivenin. I noticed her carefree attitude toward the content of her dream. She added that on another occasion she had dreamed that she was burned, "like burning at the stake." She really did not think it was so bad to be roasted. She then commented on the "funny" attitude she had toward her dreams. She announced that she was thinking about two jokes and wondered whether I wanted to hear them or not. I commented that if I said nothing, she would interpret this as my lack of interest; and if I asked about the jokes, I then might risk not taking into consideration something else she might be wanting to say. She then said the joke was about a psychiatrist who was walking down the street and one of his patients was pulling up a toothbrush by a string. The psychiatrist approached the patient and the patient told him that he was pulling this toothbrush by the string. When the psychiatrist turned his back and was a few feet away, the patient said to the toothbrush, "Hey, Joey, we really got him."

Alicia had thought that the patient in the joke did not want to tell his psychiatrist that he was hallucinating because then the psychiatrist would think the patient was crazy. She said that she was scared at night by sounds and wondered whether she was crazy herself. This session was the prelude to her first suicidal attempt two days later, but in the intervening session, she mentioned that her mother had had a course in aeronautics during the second World War and that this had been for boys, not girls.

That weekend, I received a telephone call from Alicia's father. She had been displeased with the way she looked and as the family was preparing to go to church, she had become more and more upset, refusing to attend religious services. She then had scratched her wrists with a razor blade. The father insisted on informing me about this event and requested that I see Alicia. I pointed out that if the patient wanted to see me it would be important that she call me herself. She did not call, and I saw her at our regular time two days after this episode.

During that session, Alicia was silent. When I wondered if she had any thoughts, she denied that she did. She paused again, and I asked her if she knew that her father had called me. She replied that Sunday morning she had not been pleased with her hair; she knew that her father had called because he had told her that he was going to. She had felt that she "looked awful." She had not wanted to go out and had thought of killing herself with her father's gun; but she did not have any bullets and anyhow she would not have known how to put them in. While she talked, the smile on her face was in marked contrast to the way in which her mood came through. I said that her mood conveyed the impression that she was feeling bad, not only about her hair, but about all of herself. She said that this was so, that the way she felt was "terrible." Then she expressed her annoyance because she "was yelling at herself inside for smiling." Perhaps it would be better if she died.

Her father would not have to worry about her, there would be one student less in her high school, and what would be the difference among a thousand students if one were missing? I would not need to have her as a patient; someone else would replace her. I pointed out to her that I knew she was having many bad feelings about herself, but instead of talking about them with me she had expressed them through her behavior at home. She said that her father had called me to inform me. I said that this was true, but that it was also an indirect response to something she was doing. The patient, on this occasion, was quite reluctant to talk about what had happened to her. She refused to return to the issue of her suicidal gesture and ended this particular session with protests of how her father made her feel so worthless and depreciated. She did say, nonetheless, that her mother became quite upset when she got hurt and recalled now, in the analysis, how, as a little girl, she had fallen out of the tree. When she hurt herself, I suggested, she was conveying something like wishing to hurt her father, mother, and me. She nodded. She said that she felt like hurting herself because: "Father never goes out with Mother." She would like her parents to spend more time together.

Approximately two months later, following my short absence from the office, Alicia commented on how young and little she had been only a short time ago, and how soon she would become middle-aged, old and would die. She wondered if she would not be better off dead. In fact, this had been her very first thought when she saw me. Later, in the same hour, she recalled a book that she had read. The main character died of old age, and thus was reunited with her dead beloved husband. Somehow, "to die meant to be together with those you love." She told me that she had very few friends. They either had moved away or she had lost them when she had invited them home (because they would not pay attention to her anymore afterward) or they had died. I asked her if she had had any of these thoughts while I was away. She then acknowledged that she had imagined that I was there in her room and she was talking with me. At least there was someone now, the analyst, who cared for her "half way."

Soon after, Alicia indicated that she had not changed at all in her three months of analysis and, therefore, she wanted to end her treatment. Approximately one week and a half later, she made another more serious suicidal attempt. The hour that followed (on a Friday) I shall later describe in detail; but first I shall describe the hour which preceded this more serious suicidal attempt.

Alicia began that hour as if ready to talk, but instead she became quiet the moment she had taken her seat in the chair. I interpreted to her that by not talking she was wanting very much to be in control, to prompt me to question her about what was in her mind. She responded slowly that she did not have anything important to say. She seemed quite intent on saying nothing. At times, her face wore a rather teasing, mischievous expression; at other moments, she appeared quite serious. I pointed out to her that she seemed compelled to go through these silences here, because for some reason she would rather relate to me in a way similar to the way in which she had related to her parents for many years; namely, through her behavior rather than by saying what was in her mind. At this point, near the end of the hour, Alicia was able to say, quite rapidly, what she had been thinking during her protracted silence. She had been thinking about her history class, about President Kennedy having been shot, about President Lincoln having been shot, and about the Gettysburg Address. This last reminded her of a prayer, a prayer to keep the country together. Our time was up and she said that she would be coming back for her regular session after the weekend interruption.

On Monday morning, I was informed by the social worker that the patient had slashed her wrists after an incident at the breakfast table. A younger sibling had sat in the patient's place and had refused to move. Alicia had then run upstairs and had slashed her wrists. At that moment, this sibling developed a convulsion which, for a while, diverted the parents' attention from Alicia. There had been a question of whether or not Alicia might need stitches. She had not wanted to see a surgeon because she had thought that she would thus be exposed to the world. The parents commented that, throughout the weekend, Alicia had appeared rather sulky and angry and had told them that she really hated them.

In the first session after this event, I could scarcely see Alicia's face. Her hair was combed in such a way that only a third of her face was visible as she inclined her head. She was extremely reluctant to say anything. Eventually, she said that she had cut her wrist a little deeper this time; and she had found out that her parents really did not care for her. Her father had not even insisted on her seeing a physician. But, she added, it made no difference because even though she now would have an ugly scar, she had another ugly scar on her face anyhow—a scar that she had "not even done anything to get." Nobody cared for her, not even she, herself. She did not think she was going to change. Again, she protested that she was disappointed in her analysis. When she had started analysis, she had hoped for something, she did not know exactly what, but now she was wasting her time, my time, and her father's money. Any discussion of the suicidal attempt she dropped quite skillfully. She stressed her feeling of being pushed by her parents, wondered to what extent she was commited to the treatment situation, how much part she had in determining whether she was in treatment or not, and so on. At that point, I inadvertently went along with this avoidance.

Alicia missed two sessions and then returned. On this occasion she was silent for most of the hour. I reminded her of what had happened over the weekend and how she had felt so unable to express her feelings either to her parents or to me, and how instead she had felt compelled to slash her wrist. In response, she said that she was afraid I would laugh at her. A typical defensive device she used was to reverse roles: for example, to emphasize what I was doing to her instead of what she had been doing to me.

One week later, she stated that she had felt depressed the previous weekend, and that this weekend she was feeling so happy. She said that over the weekend she talks "with the other Doctor K." She tells this other doctor all the "stuff that bugs her." I commented that she had constructed a Doctor K all for herself, but a doctor that neither answered back nor helped her in reality except by being present in accordance with her wishes and by giving her the illusion that everything was fine. The fantasied Doctor K, I added, had certainly proved insufficient to help with the problem that she had been going through the previous weekend.

In the following months, Alicia made isolated references to her suicidal tendencies. At one point, she said that she felt her parents' work with the social worker, and the social worker's contact with the analyst, indicated that we were all members of a conspiracy designed to make her "angry and mad," so that she would "end up by wanting to kill" herself. She said this in a rather teasing, smiling tone. She added that this was rather silly, to have "lumped all of us together" in this way.

A frequently repeated statement which Alicia made in the context of separations and disappointments may shed light on the omnipotence fantasies connected with her suicidal acts: namely, that whenever she was in a good mood, nothing bad could happen to her. At times, she felt "so good" that "if my house were on fire, or if I had killed myself, or if I had been robbed of my money, this would not affect me."

On one occasion, she told a story about a giant called Mighty Pee. This was a small giant who could accomplish great things. He could really move mountains. Perhaps this applied to herself, she said. She was a small person and had wanted to accomplish a lot of things, too. She would like to be a child psychologist, or a child psychiatrist; but not a pediatrician because she could not stand children's deaths. She paused. When I inquired about what she was thinking, she said she was remembering a hymn in her church. She then imagined herself alone in an apartment with someone ringing the bell; she opened the door and was shot. I suggested that there would be something dangerous for this "little person" were she to attain fulfillment of her wishes.

A few months later, suicidal themes receded and gave way instead to Alicia's anxieties about bodily harm, or destructive wishes directed against parts of her own body. She acknowledged "it was funny" that she was so afraid of cutting her face, or having a pin stuck in her eye. She recalled that one summer, when she was leaving her job, she saw some broken glass on the street. The thought had occurred to her that were she to fall she would be quite fearful of cutting her face. She was also afraid of cutting her arm, she said, but "if you cut your arms, you can still cover them, but on the face it is much worse." She paused briefly and said "it was funny" that on the one hand she was so afraid she might cut herself, yet, on the other hand, she had deliberately cut her wrist. Indeed, she was always afraid that an accident might occur and that she might cut her face. Later in the hour, she stated for the first time that when the obstetrician had hurt her face, he had "done this on purpose." At that moment, she started to prick herself with a pin which she was holding. I interpreted this action as her way of saying that if she pricked herself, at least it was she, herself, who was doing it and she was not being taken by surprise, unprepared and defenseless as she had been when she was born.[3] Alicia experienced intense hatred of her body. She used to comment on how she felt she had really a "bad face, a thousand miles long," ugly fingers, short nails, and ugly legs. I commented that she seemed to refer only to the periphery of her body and made no mention of her trunk. She looked at me and said that the human being is an ugly animal. I wondered whether she thought the bodies of boys and girls were equally ugly. She thought that they were. She believed that the physiology of the human body was "marvelous" but that the "outside was awful." While talking with me, she was trying to prick open a blister on her hand. She said that this would not harm her; she was not bothered by the sight of blood. I asked her if she had a different feeling about the blood of her menstrual periods. She immediately acknowledged that this really did bother her. She found herself ugly enough with the scar on her face. I wondered if perhaps she had thought that her genitals also represented some scar, some kind of wound that bleeds once a month, and that she had felt there was no hope of ever changing that. Now she became quite reflective and serious and said, rather shyly, that she did feel like that. She had also felt like having an operation to rid herself of her sense of physical damage. Rather reluctantly, she referred to "some operations" in which "you take the ovary and the uterus from the woman, so you change the woman to nothing." Thus, she would not have to bear children nor would she bleed. With her characteristic reversal of affect, she added that it was fun to think about such an operation.

By the fifth month of analysis, the transference neurosis had developed quite fully, as illustrated by the following excerpt: After a pause, I asked Alicia if she had any thoughts. For a month, now, the hours had been characterized by long silences. I had told her that I had noticed that these silences had changed their nature, and I had encouraged her to observe them and sort them out and see what they meant. She said perhaps I could tell her what the silence implied because I was smarter than she. I responded by saying that sometimes she felt the opposite. She then mentioned that she was thinking about "another thing"; she would have her teeth pulled. She hoped her own dentist would do this and not refer her to someone else. She really "doesn't want a stranger to run out with her teeth." Her doctor would have to give her anesthesia; it might very well be that she was allergic also to Novocain and that she could have a rough time. I then said that her fear of the dentist pulling her teeth reminded me of how she had told me that she was afraid here of "losing her philosophy." If the dentist got into her mouth, or if I got into her mind, she might lose something that she really cherished, as though I would destroy something in her. Rather subdued, she looked at me, and conveyed the impression that she had, indeed, lost something right there and then. I shared this impression with her, telling her that she looked as if she had the vague feeling of having lost something at that moment, and as if she were afraid this might happen again here. She then complained that her fourth and fifth fingers and half of her right forearm were numb. Laughingly, she said, "If I had my fingers amputated, it wouldn't hurt now." She said that her fingers had felt numb last week, too, and this always happened right here in the sessions. Sometimes her legs, also, would grow numb when she pressed on them.

Information about Alicia's family, conveyed by the caseworker at this time, indicated that the patient appeared more relaxed, was involved in more peer activities, dressed more fashionably, had lost weight, and had not recently engaged in outbursts with her parents.

During the second year of analysis, we worked intensively on Alicia's aggressive impulses and her guilt in relation to masturbatory activities and fantasies.

She had been reading *I Never Promised You a Rose Garden*. At one point, I wondered if, because she wanted to steal some of my possessions, my patients, my job, she were afraid that I might want to do the same to her. She then said that perhaps she was like the patient in the book who was afraid of poisoning the therapist with her words. She suggested that I read the book and then I would know what had happened. I said that she wanted me to know her through the book and not directly; perhaps this was an attempt to protect me from her poison. She sighed and said that she had really liked this book; "to tell the truth," at one point, when reading it, she had felt like slashing her wrists, but she then had felt that she could not do this. Simultaneously, she had felt like holding someone's hand and like crying. The patient in the book had had a relapse, and she was now in the middle of reading about this. She was sure that the patient would eventually get better.

During the next few months of this second analytic year, Alicia's narcissistic character defenses, with omnipotent fantasies of control of her fate, revealed a new and important layer of her suicidal fantasies. Thus, in her fantasies, she played herself against fate in order to control it. If some future event, which she wished very much to happen, seemed really uncertain, she would characteristically say, "I'm going to kill myself if this does not happen." She even set deadlines for taking an overdosage of pills.

In this period, Alicia experienced guilt about sexual play with her brother and for having watched her father in the nude. She felt that her childhood sexual activities had ruined her life. She wanted to return to her childhood, and she thought of the Garden of Eden where everything was pure.

She felt sad for some days. She recalled Andersen's story of the little mermaid who had given up her most valuable possession, her voice, so that she could be with her beloved prince. She could not talk to him, however, and finally realized that he was fond of someone else and that "they were made for each other." The little mermaid then returned to the sea and did many good deeds before going to Heaven. But, did she go to Heaven? Alicia did not exactly remember the end of the story. On another occasion, as she was examining her attachment to her father, she declared that she felt so guilty that she thought she should die. She equated her close relationship to her father with adultery, which was sinful. Since "right now every boy represents my dad, that is why I cannot marry or date—the only solution is to die."

An interruption of the analysis over Christmas vacation brought up the following feelings: Alicia insisted that she had "to break the tie." She was going to leave *me*; and she told me that she was expecting to have a date for the holiday season and to go to a party. I commented how frightened she was to let me know that she thought of having a good time when I would be away. I suggested to her that it was as though I would envy her were she to have a nice time, just as she envied me my going away. She said bitterly that I was such an exceptional person; I had everything, family and profession. She wanted to terminate analysis. I wondered if she wanted to terminate treatment because she would like to keep some good things before I spoiled them for her, just as she would like to spoil my good things because she envied my having everything. Terminating treatment and becoming her own psychiatrist were efforts geared toward having no envy of me. She sighed and said that sometimes she felt like a "leech"; she added that she might catch pneumonia and die during my absence, or drive her car into a pole. I said that this "leechy" feeling made her feel so bad that she felt like paying for it by having pneumonia or an accident. This was the last day before Christmas vacation, and she wished me a Merry Christmas which I reciprocated.

Two years after the initiation of her treatment, Alicia announced her intention to spend a summer in Europe. She stated her plans, however, in terms of asking me directly whether she should go; and, as an expression of her anger, she announced that she was not going to return after the first of the year, because she needed to be on her own. Immediately following this session, I became ill. While I was at home, the patient called to tell me that she was feeling depressed; she was thinking of killing herself and had already taken one Compazine pill. She indeed sounded depressed; it had not been her pattern to call me. I found it difficult to continue exploring the problem on the phone, and I said that I hoped I would be back in the office at the first of the coming week. Did she think she could wait until then? She did not know, she said; she might not be alive the following day. I suggested that I could arrange for someone to see her if she felt it was too much for her to wait. She said she might want to do that; however, she also might want to go for a walk and perhaps that would help. I suggested that she could phone me the following morning and let me know.

When the patient called me the next morning, she sounded much less depressed. She told me she had had a dream:

> She was swimming on a cloudy day. Someone was attempting to shoot at her, and she cried, "Doctor Paul, Doctor Paul." There was a face that appeared and disappeared. Finally she climbed over a rock and felt like a wet rat.

I listened to Alicia's dream. However, as we were talking on the phone, I asked her only how she understood her feelings. She said she did not know. I reminded her of her habit of analyzing some of her thoughts and dreams on her own. I also reminded her that her having asked me for approval for her trip abroad sounded like her plans the previous summer when she also had asked me if she could go to the West Coast, as though sometimes she wanted to leave the responsibility for herself to me or to her parents. She then replied ironically that "an analyst always lets you know that your life is your own life, that your decisions are your own decisions, and that your suicide is your own suicide." She terminated the conversation rather angrily.

The following session, the patient reproached me for having been sick. She said, "I became so upset that I fouled the whole thing up" (the trip to Europe). She then retold the dream she had mentioned on the phone. I wondered whether her dream could help us understand what might have contributed to her despondency. She said that in the dream she had felt like "being born in the sea." Someone had been shooting at her, perhaps she had been shooting at herself because of her sins, or had her father shot at her? She remembered that a few years earlier she had wanted to shoot herself but had not been able to find a gun around the house. She then associated to "Paul." She had a cousin who had a very destructive brother, Paul, who built models and then destroyed them. I wondered about the relation of Paul to Paulina (the analyst's name). "Paulina is the masculine of Paul," she said. I wondered about Paulina being the masculine of Paul. "Ha," she said, "I meant feminine." Her association to "feeling like a wet rat," was that Paul, who used to tease her, was a rat. She added that the fairy godmother in Cinderella turned rats into coachmen. She thought of rats as being voracious, snatching cookies from the hands of sleeping children in slum neighborhoods.

I reminded Alicia that when she had first told me of the dream on the telephone, she had said she was calling for "Doctor Paul." I commented on the relationship between her feeling abandoned by me because of my absence, and this Doctor Paul who appeared and disappeared in the dream, and her thoughts of going abroad and terminating her treatment. I suggested that she felt depressed because she felt that she had to give me up, and to give up the illusion that I was Paul and not Paulina, and that she herself was a girl and not a damaged boy. I suggested that she also felt she had to give up the hope that, like the fairy godmother, I would transform her from a "voracious wet rat" into a coachman, a man. I suggested that her suicidal threats represented an effort to force me to give her advice about the trip, pills, anything.

Alicia sighed and said she had forgotten to mention that during those days of my absence, she had thought about having a hysterectomy. She had started her period and she hated her menstruation. She felt quite guilty to find herself so demanding of me and she thought it was terrible to feel so greedy and voracious. Near the end of the hour, she returned to the theme of the trip. "You don't have objections to my going then; this means I can go. It also means that I am not ready to quit; I have to analyze this thing."

Further work on her telephone call and her suicidal intentions could now be achieved. Alicia had felt abandoned when she most needed me, and her phoning me to tell me how bad she felt was a way of reproaching me. She added, "You didn't even give me pills." I asked her what came to mind about getting pills and she replied that pills were white and convex. She wanted to get all of these pills and have it over with. I wondered if she had called me not only to convey how desperate she felt, but also to convey that if she were not permitted to go abroad, she would become as demanding as a little child because this was how she felt she was being treated. She had interpreted my absence, after she had told me about Europe, and my refusal to tell her to go there, as an actual prohibition against the trip. When I suggested that she would demand these white convex pills as a child would demand the breast or the bottle, she started to cry, trying to control her tears with anxious giggling.

The patient's guilt feelings regarding her masturbatory experiences, her competitiveness, and her jealousy were very intense. "You never mentioned my good qualities," she said, "the dirty stuff only." Alicia complained that in two and a half years of analysis she had not gained self-esteem. She became provocative, trying to control me with cutting remarks. Her anger, when she discovered unacceptable aspects of herself, could only be expressed by thoughts of killing herself, thus conveying the impression that she was punishing herself. She said that she had hated herself when she had started treatment. If I had just looked at her, I would have known. She used to think that I hated her, but now she felt that I had made her hate herself. She said with great sarcasm and bitterness, "You have done this for me, you have done a mighty fine job." She succeeded in making me experience a sense of exasperation and futility.

Almost every day thereafter, Alicia would give hints of suicidal threats. She would include her suicidal thoughts as part of a barrage of attacks against me. Frequently she would say that she felt bad and undeserving of love. She felt like killing herself now with rum and pills. She said that she felt so sinful as a result of all the things she had learned about herself in her analysis that, once dead, she would certainly go to Heaven. In Heaven, God would review her life and would think that she was not so bad, but He, God, would be mistaken.

Alicia now thought that she would kill herself on the anniversary of the death of a close relative. "I am no good—my birth was a mistake." "Actually," she went on, "it is not my fault that I was conceived and born, nor that I have feelings of jealousy." This was the prelude to her first talk in detail about her masturbatory practices. The patient had unfolded the theme of masturbation with great difficulty throughout her analysis. During the first year, she had made only nonverbal references to masturbation. For example, she would hide her hands consistently behind her purse. Now, she admitted painfully that she used a flashlight, a gift from a paternal uncle, and castigated herself by slapping her face while making this admission.

Alicia expressed surprise that I did not react to her confession by hitting her. She said she felt dirty, no good. Her father would beat her up if he knew about her masturbation. Later, she thought more about the ''flashlight.'' She associated light with something burning hot, which might hurt and leave a wound. When masturbating, she had made herself bleed, and she did not know how much harm she had done to herself. We now understood the meaning of her suicidal gestures early in her analysis.

Her envy of the parental couple, and the realization that she would eventually have to be on her own, brought up much hostility. Thoughts of suicide to protect her good objects from her destructiveness emerged. She thought of how time passed and of how her parents' neighborhood had started to deteriorate, and of her house crumbling. She felt like dying right then, during the hour. I pointed out that she was thinking of death to protect me and her parents from her badness. She said that she had already killed herself psychically, but not yet physically. The confrontation with her unacceptable aggressive wishes enraged her.

Alicia thought of her impending funeral. I would be there and, out of happiness for having got rid of the patient, I would pat myself so hard on the shoulder that I would fracture my arm. I commented on her wish to hurt me or harm me under the guise of being, herself, already dead. She said that I had given her all the understanding she needed to feel poorly; I had never told her that I was glad about any of her good qualities.

During the ensuing period, the patient conveyed the feeling of having destroyed everything good that she, herself, had admitted the analysis had given her. She stated repeatedly that she had only one week left in which to live. She was going to kill herself because she was undeserving of love. She would die as criminals die, by electrocution or by hanging. I pointed out to her that every day she was threatening me with her thoughts of dying, attacking me for my failure to help her, while, at the same time, she was reproaching me for my mistreatment of her. I said that her self-disparaging thoughts protected her from feeling guilty about her attacks on me. She cried and said that her relative had died at this time of year and that she had killed her because she hated her. How could I, her analyst, love her if she were so unworthy? Now I knew all the bad things about her. If she were left on her own, she would feel compelled to punish herself by suicide.

For what seemed to me endless sessions, Alicia became increasingly vehement in her suicidal threats. I suggested that if she felt unable to manage her impulses, she could be hospitalized. She promptly responded that I would not be willing to hospitalize her, because I did not care enough. I pointed out that if she could not handle this, we would need to let her parents know, so that she would not hurt herself. But we would still need to continue the working through of her feelings. She then threatened me by saying that maybe she would kill herself that same day! I said firmly that if she could not bear this thought without having to act upon it, I would not hesitate to take steps which would prevent her from hurting herself.

The following session, Alicia told me that she was surprised she had come to this hour. "Yesterday [Sunday], I was home alone and thought of how convenient a time it was to kill myself. I thought I would take pills, but then I would have to have my stomach pumped and go to the hospital as a 'suicidal attempt.' Besides, I did not like writing a suicide note." I commented that she had been thinking every day about what to do with her feelings of resentment, envy, hatefulness, and demandingness; the only way that she could express these feelings was by repeating to me her thoughts of suicide and by seeing herself as my victim. However, I added, at this point we needed to clarify whether she could contain these fantasies or whether she needed hospitalization because she felt driven to act upon these feelings. She said that she should drown herself. Here again, I confronted her with the fact that she admitted her hostility only when she was simultaneously attacking herself as she now was doing with her thoughts of drowning. At this moment, she made a slip. Instead of saying that she would kill herself, she said, she would "kill themselves." She described herself as "feeling in a fog." She thought that she would end her life the next weekend. Bitterly, she said, "If you fall in love and you get married, you act upon your feelings. If you want to study, you act upon your feelings. If you want to commit suicide, you act upon those feelings, too." Then reluctantly, Alicia said that she would have to miss college were she to hospitalize herself, and the hospital might be too expensive. Confronted with the possible consequences of her threats, she ended the hour with a "damn it."

Here, there was a crucial issue at stake: The patient's acceptance of herself as a girl, that is, of her genital feminine passivity, without regressing to oral-dependent needs. This was a particularly difficult task owing to her marked oral fixations. Progressively, Alicia began to postpone her intended suicide to the future. She would kill herself after graduating from college, or at any other time were she to feel frustrated and find life too painful or difficult for her. Near termination, she recalled my having been supportive of her as an inconsistency in my technique. "You had grown hysterical like me, when I was threatening suicide." She had noticed this because I had "talked too much," a realistic perception of my own anxiety as expressed in my suggestion of hospitalization.

The beginning of the third year of treatment was a most difficult period for Alicia. She became increasingly demanding while continuing to threaten me with suicide. At the same time, she continued to work on her masturbation problem. In the transference, I became a sadistic persecutor who forced her to talk about these terrible things (masturbation). She described her masturbation fantasies in a more detailed way and finally, with great effort, talked of her conviction that by masturbating she had actually hurt herself irreparably. She felt hopeless and thought that nobody could erase the damage that she had caused herself.

In the past, she said that she felt so hurt, so disqualified when she had to think about how dependent and demanding she was, that the only solution she found was to kill herself. At that time, I interpreted this in terms of her attempts to control the analysis of these aspects of herself. Now suicidal threats also occurred when she realized that she depended on me, and when she could not control my coming and going either during vacations or because of illness. I happened to be ill on occasions when she was in the midst of working through her attacks on her introjected objects. She became very anxious when I was not available, and my absence made it more difficult for her to resolve her omnipotence fantasies regarding the damaging effects on me of her aggressiveness. In fact, after my most recent absence, she had considered not returning to treatment.

At one point, Alicia raised the question of whether I thought that she might kill herself. I pointed out to her that she was putting me in the position of an oracle. In the past, I said, she had asked me when she could terminate, whether she should become a psychiatrist, and now she was asking if she were able to kill herself. She burst into a series of reproaches: I was not helping her; maybe she should get another psychiatrist; it was "not getting through my thick skull and small brains" that she really did not want an answer but only wanted to be helped to find one. I replied that, on the one hand, she was putting me on a pedestal like an oracle (she giggled and said like the sphinx in Thebes), and, on the other hand, she was telling me that I was not worth listening to, that I had a thick skull and small brains. She became rather disconcerted, started to talk about her troubles in school, and then asked me whether she could become a psychiatrist. When no answer was forthcoming, she said that she could be anything she wanted, and that I did not care about what she was going to be. She could become a psychiatrist or a nurse. She could become a prostitute or, after all, she could kill herself. I would even encourage her to end her life; I would not care about what she did. I told her that she was expecting me to react and to tell her definitely what my stand was. She expected me to be like a parent who would approve or support or comfort her and, because I would not comply, she was quite angry and she threatened to kill herself, which would serve me right. Alicia repeatedly discarded or opposed these comments.

Later, she talked about termination. She associated this with the death of the relationship between her and me. She said she was afraid of what was to come, and that I was the only person who accepted her. I wondered if she were afraid that, were she to be left on her own, she would be a victim of her own destructive, bad feelings. She then said that there was one word which she experienced constantly when thinking about herself and this was "hate." She also said that, although she knew termination would cause neither herself nor me to die, the relationship would die—she would never see me again. She had thoughts about a boa constrictor clutching her, stifling her. With a nervous giggle, she said, "Who knows? I might be eaten up and swallowed by a boa constrictor." She indicated thus her efforts to rid herself of the mother-introject. So strong was the link that separation threatened the survival of either one of the pair.

Meantime, Alicia was proceeding with her plans to go abroad on her vacation.

In one of our most stormy sessions, as she continued to consider termination, she was associating about getting old, being alone, and death. At this very moment, she had a "funny" sensation, a spinning feeling as though she were going to lose her equilibrium. I said this was what termination and going away meant to her: being out of control and powerless. She compared herself with a turtle who was leaving her shell. What would a turtle out of the shell look like? To be lying on the couch was to be like a turtle turned on its back, defenseless; the analyst might take out her eyes, hit her, cut her. She then repeated her accusation that I did not care whether she died or not. She bitterly reproached me for the fact that when she had slashed her wrist, I had merely said that, if she wanted to see me, I could see her the following day. I had never hospitalized her. What kind of doctor was I? If a patient broke her leg, would the doctor just order the patient to walk? If she decided she was going to be a prostitute, or to commit suicide, I would not even protect her. I commented that it was quite painful for her to be faced with the fact that she still hoped to find in me a powerful parent who could save her from all uncertainties. And because she also was aware that I would not fulfill that role, she was so enraged and expressed this rage by thoughts of killing herself. It had been most painful for her to learn, throughout her treatment, that she was not a powerful giant, nor was I.

In the following session, the patient said that I had hurt her tremendously. She had thought of killing herself the previous night. She might die one of these days; and she had come to the conclusion that I did not care for her, that I was an incompetent physician who did not help my patients, and that I would most certainly become involved in a malpractice law suit. She said she was furious, repeating this several times throughout the hour. She was going to write a note to her parents, stating that they had been good parents, and that they were not at fault. To die was her own responsibility. Her implication was that I had conveyed to her that what she wanted to do with herself was her own responsibility. She wished to write this suicidal note, in which she would state that it was all my fault, and this would initiate a malpractice law suit. She was going to kill herself because I had hurt her, because I did not care for her, and because she was just an ugly duckling.

I pointed out to Alicia that her threats of suicide were an effort to protect herself from what she thought was my impending attack on her. She feared, I said, that I would retaliate for her feeling so aggressive, for her trying to destroy my reputation by a malpractice law suit. She protested that I was the one who hated her. I said that she needed very much to see me as hating her because at least this would make her feel less bad about herself. If she hated me, but I also hated her, she would not have to feel so guilty. She then thought that she was going to die. She was going to take pills. I said that this was another way in which to kill and destroy me, to destroy me inside of herself. This was the way she had felt about her parents when she had slashed her wrists.

Alicia said on many occasions that I should let her terminate her treatment or recommend her to another psychiatrist because of her threats to kill herself. I conveyed to her that she was leaving it up to me to finish her treatment or to send her away to another psychiatrist because she was afraid of my retaliation for her leaving me and for her wanting to attack me with a malpractice law suit. She said that her hatred was so intense it was unbearable. She felt she was full of "meanies," and proceeded to describe vividly a world of devilish creatures of all colors and shapes. Because she had become so demanding, she was afraid that I could not stand it and that I would have to tell somebody how she made me suffer. I added that perhaps she dreaded I would tell my husband and yet also wished he would disagree with me about her, a situation rather like the one which she had created with her parents. Paradoxically, the parents now had united against her and she felt more deprived than ever because mother and father stood together while she was left out. As I was telling her this, she said her body felt "funny." She was quite dizzy, as though she were dying. She was not sure whether she could move or walk. She started to say to herself, "control yourself, you will be all right, you will come out of this room and go to your classes, and nobody will know that anything happened."

In a later session, Alicia compared her illness to a tumor in her head. Maybe her illness was incurable. At lunchtime that day, her mother had told her that when she was born her milk had "run out," and that when Alicia was a few weeks old she had been very hungry. At first, the mother had not known what was happening, but finally she had realized that Alicia was hungry and she had given her her formula. Alicia said that seemed still to be happening to her: "I am always looking for the real thing, no substitute is enough." I said to her that she now felt that she was not being gratified by me and therefore she had to destroy whatever she did receive and thus she felt more dissatisfied. She was notably sad during this hour and cried.

Alicia now developed some concern for me. She thought that were she to kill herself because she was not feeling any better about what she had found out in her analysis, she would do so only after treatment had terminated. In that case, her parents might or might not file a malpractice suit against me, and I could defend myself on the grounds that it had not been clear that she would commit suicide. It was interesting that the moment she experienced some concern about the way in which her feelings were affecting me, she ceased her suicidal threats.

Summer was approaching and she wondered if she would want to terminate treatment when she returned from abroad. She expressed her wish not to die a spinster. She would hate to have "Gone, but not forgotten" as an epitaph. Indeed, we had worked through to a great extent, the sadomasochistic implications for her of the primal scene. She now acknowledged that her analysis was helping her to undo the internal block she had carried for many years.

In the fall, Alicia returned from her trip abroad. She had had a most successful vacation. For the first time, she seemed to face the world on her own without experiencing the ominous forebodings of the past.

As she had intended to do many months earlier, she decreased progressively the frequency of her hours, in spite of my active efforts to prevent this decision by interpretation. We explored the various underlying meanings of her plan, including the "weaning" implication; her fear and wish that I would not survive after her departure, so that her one weekly session would serve the purpose of reassuring her that I was alive and did not hate her. We also explored her fantasy that her coming on a once-a-week basis would render our relationship "friendlier." At this time, she had the following dream:

> There were many dead people in a mausoleum. She was going downstairs into another chamber, at the door of which stood the man who takes care of the material for the college laboratory. She saw a box, rather a grave, and she was afraid she would be locked in there. She told this to the man at the door, and he responded, "This is a wish that many people here have. . . ."

Alicia was so frightened by this dream that she woke up. The previous night she had been thinking of killing herself. She feared that, like a friend of hers who, after many years of treatment, still could not hold a job or study, she also would not be able to function on her own. At this point, her ambivalence about termination could be dealt with. She could now realistically accept my function by arriving at the definition of an analyst as one who "lets you solve your own problems by talking, without hospitalization and drugs."

Only three months of treatment remained. Another wave of suicidal threats developed when Alicia "discovered" that I was expecting a baby. She was the last of my patients to make this observation verbally explicit in the treatment. Although I knew she had learned of my pregnancy from a third person a fortnight earlier, she acknowledged her awareness only by threatening suicide. "I want to do away with myself because I am undeserving of love." She had too much to do, she had already tasted a little bit of life on her trip abroad, and she had tasted enough so she now could die; and thus, she said, another patient could replace her.

I interpreted this material as a reflection of her envy of my baby and linked this interpretation to her longings to stay with me for an indefinite period. Now, in the transference, Alicia's renewed suicidal threats clearly expressed a sadistic attack on the mother, which was related to her sibling rivalry. Until this time, she had repressed the full impact of the birth of her siblings.

In the next session, one week later, Alicia spoke of her plans for the future. At the beginning of the hour, she said that I might as well sit down so that I would not get too tired. This was her first direct acknowledgment of my pregnancy. I wondered whether her comment had to do with her having noticed changes in my appearance; she smiled and said, "You certainly are expecting a baby!" She then added: "I lead my life, I go my way, and you go yours." I remarked on her insistence that this was none of her business. She replied, without much conviction, that I was so important. However, she was only coming once a week now and had many other problems on her mind.

We still had several sessions before I was due to begin my maternity leave. The patient again decided that this was going to be her last hour. "It was really unfair," she said, that I had not let her know more in advance that I was to be away; I must have known when I was going to have the baby. She complained that I had been mistreating her and that she had so few opportunities in which to talk with me. I pointed out that she had insisted on reducing the frequency of hours to once a week. She then complained that I also had mistreated her by never having hospitalized her. I said that she was very angry because she had not been able to control me and to force me to do what she wanted (hospitalization, support, counseling, pills, and so forth). I suggested that her most intense anger over her failure to control me was related to her awareness of my pregnancy: she could not tolerate, she thought, her intense envy of my baby and of me. She began to cry. She knew she had to live with her envy as well as with her masturbation, but this was very painful and hard for her. This session marked a turning point toward the resolution of her suicidal fantasies.

Upon my return two months later, Alicia sent me a message

informing me that she was going to adhere to her decision to terminate. The following excerpts are from a letter I received:

I appreciate your concern very much, but I must stick to my decision. I promised myself not to set foot into another psychiatrist's office after the next year and promises are not to be broken. . . .

I guess the first thing I'll do is to assure you I'm getting along fine. I've stuck by my decision to go to [a college in a neighboring town]. I went with my friend; we walked around on campus for awhile and talked with the college staff. . . .

I hope you can understand, but nothing, not even psychoanalysis, can go on forever. There always comes a time to say goodbye. Sometimes it is very painful to say goodbye to someone and know you'll never see them again the rest of your life. Sometimes it hurts like *hell*, but it is part of life and it just has to be accepted as such! If I came back now, it would only hurt more to say goodbye later and I really don't think I can stand it. Please understand this and accept my decision. I know you are only my psychoanalyst, but I also consider you my friend.

Before I sign off, I must say "Thank you, thank you very much!" I really appreciate all you have done for me and please accept my thanks. God bless you.

Alicia.

After this letter, I phoned Alicia to ask her to come in for what proved to be her last session. She arrived with a new, fashionable hair-do and dressed in a typical college outfit. She had agreed to come because she wanted to see me again, and also because I had insisted she come and talk with me. Also, she wanted to tell me that she was not coming any more! She was definitely going to terminate treatment. She wanted me to accept her decision and to wait and see how she did on her own in the future. She would let me know if she were having problems, or even if she were not having them.

She had thought about why I had left her without giving her sufficient notice. First, she had thought I wanted to make her feel so angry about my sudden departure that she would have to continue treatment. Later, she thought maybe I might not have known exactly when I was going to have to leave, something must have come up at the last moment and I could not help it. It was this latter thought which made her decide to come to this hour and to "give me a chance." She asked me what really had happened.

I said that what impressed me most was her readiness to experience me as a bad person, somebody who could make things intolerable for her. I wondered if right now she also might be thinking that, should I respect her decision to terminate in this particular way, this would mean that I was glad to be rid of her! No sooner had I said this, when she asked me quite candidly, "Well, aren't you getting rid of me?" and then she laughed. She explained that were she to have any future doubts about having ended the analysis, it would be important to have me available; and she asked me not to be "mad at her" because she was terminating. She said that this was also like leaving one's parents. It was possible to leave them if they did not say "don't ever come again." This had happened to one of her girl friends who had been married the previous December, and whose parents were not completely in accord with their daughter's choice of a husband yet were still willing to accept her. That was important because "if you have troubles, then you have a family to talk to." Lastly, she did not want to become a psychiatrist, because there was a high incidence of suicide among psychiatrists; and women psychiatrists committed suicide more than did men psychiatrists. For a person such as herself, who had suicidal tendencies, "it would be suicide to choose such a profession!" She ended by affirming the fact that she had learned to enjoy life, to be a human being, and that she now preferred the Jewish religion because Jews did not accept the idea of the original sin.

DISCUSSION

Although I have selected the theme of suicide for this paper, the outcome of the treatment was favorable. The patient had improved considerably in her symptomatic, characterological, and social adjustment. Her self-esteem had risen, she had begun to date, she had become more hopeful about the future. Her appearance had changed to that of a bright young lady, attractively dressed. Her obesity and allergies had all but disappeared. Her basic characterological features, a mixture of hysterical, compulsive, and narcissistic traits were attenuated and had lost their rigidity.[4]

Alicia's suicidal threats were directed against multiple targets within the self: (1) against object representations reflecting sadistic introjected parental images (especially the parents united in sexual intercourse, and perceived sadistically as a result of the projection of her own jealousy and envy onto them); (2) against self-representations, reflecting her guilt arising from the positive and negative oedipal wishes which were connected with her sexual excitement (hurting herself as a punishment for her sexual impulses as well as a disguised gratification of them); and (3) against her body image, which was utilized as a symbolic representation of her genitals (fantasies of bodily mutilation represented regressive, sadomasochistic masturbatory fantasies in both form and content).

Alicia's suicidal threats also served multiple instinctual and defensive needs in the transference. Thus, her oral greediness and demandingness were acted out in the transference in her attempts to force me to submit to her requests for unlimited gratification. Her suicidal threats also reflected the activation of primitive omnipotence and control as defensive operations aimed toward protecting her narcissistic features which she exposed in the transference. In this regard, suicide represented the ultimate independence from the depreciation of, an impinging, hostile external world. In more general terms, suicidal threats provided the patient with control over her parents, interference with their intimacy, and ongoing overinvolvement with them.

Suicidal threats and fantasies, serving all of the above-mentioned needs, shifted throughout the treatment for the purpose both of defense against, and expression of, her struggles around her feminine sexual identity. Masturbatory fantasies and actions were successfully avoided by the creation of her several suicidal attempts as well as by her repeated suicidal threats. The types of suicidal action envisioned by the patient reflected her changing images of herself as a woman: from the fantasies of shooting herself with a gun (a masculine suicidal fantasy formation) she shifted to fantasies of ingesting pills (a more typical feminine suicidal fantasy).

Against these developments on a genital and oedipal level, defensive regression to primitive oral conflicts were reactivated, over and over, and here again took the form of suicidal fantasies. To die meant for her to return to paradise, the ultimate source of primitive gratification; it also represented the expiation of her guilt feelings arising from her greediness and demandingness. Above all, suicidal threats permitted her the expression of violent depreciation and devaluation of the analyst as a frustrating source of help.

Envy of the analyst's work, to the point of the patient's hating her own improvement because it confirmed the value of the envied analyst, was vividly expressed as suicidal threats which stressed her hopelessness and the lack of help she received from the analyst. At the same time, suicide was seen by the patient as a protection against retaliation by the transference object whom she had attacked.

One might speculate to what extent, in times of severe regression, fusion of self and object images may have complicated the functions of Alicia's suicidal fantasies, so that attacks on her self-representations were indistinguishable from efforts to extricate herself from engulfing, bad internal objects (represented, for example, by fantasies such as that of the boa constrictor). As the treatment proceeded, her concern about herself increased together with her growing realistic awareness and control of her behavior. Her tendency to act upon her suicidal wishes and fantasies gradually decreased and, as suicidal action disappeared, the unfolding meanings of the fantasies could be increasingly contained within the treatment situation.

NOTES

[1] According to Seiden (1969), boys more frequently attempt suicide by gunshot or by means of rope hanging, whereas girls more typically make suicidal attempts with pills or some other toxic material.

[2] At the Menninger Foundation, the parents of children and most adolescents in psychoanalysis are currently in casework with a social worker. I am aware that this team approach is not necessarily standard practice elsewhere.

[3] It was only many months later that my knowledge of Alicia's masturbatory activities enabled me to understand what she said immediately afterward: "It is better for me to hurt myself because I am not in danger of hurting myself badly." In fact her masturbatory activities consisted of self-stimulation with a flashlight which had been given to her by her father, and which she occasionally would use so vigorously as to induce slight bleeding.

[4] In spite of the gains she derived from the treatment, she did not work through sufficiently such aspects of her termination as her fear of her homosexual attachment to me and her belief that by breaking her ties to me she could break her ties to her parents, all of which factors had contributed to her need to end her analysis prematurely.

BIBLIOGRAPHY

Balser, B.H., and Masterson, J.F., Jr. 1959. Suicide in adolescents. *American Journal of Psychiatry* 116:400-404.

Barter, J.T., Swaback, D.O., and Todd, D. 1968. Adolescent suicide attempts. *Archives of General Psychiatry* 19:523-27.

Farberow, N.L. 1961. Summary. In *The cry for help*, ed. N.L. Farberow and E.S. Shneidman, pp. 290-321. New York: McGraw-Hill.

Geleerd, E.R. 1961. Some aspects of ego vicissitudes in adolescence. *Journal of the American Psychoanalytic Association* 9:394-405.

Gould, R.E. 1965. Suicide problems in children and adolescents. *American Journal of Psychotherapy* 19:228-46.

Greenacre, P. 1950. Special problems of early female sexual development. *Psychoanalytic Study of the Child* 5:122-38.

———. 1952a. Prepuberty trauma in girls. In *Trauma, growth and personality*, pp. 204-33. New York: W.W. Norton.

———. 1952b. Some factors producing different types of genital and pregenital organization. In *Trauma, growth and personality*, pp. 293-302. New York: W. W. Norton.

Harley, M. 1961a. Masturbation conflicts. In *Adolescents: Psychoanalytic approach to problems and therapy*, ed. S. Lorand and H. Schneer, pp. 51-77. New York: Hoeber.

———. 1961b. Some observations on the relationship between genitality and structural development at adolescence. *Journal of the American Psychoanalytic Association* 9:434-60.

Hendin, H. 1961. Suicide: A psychoanalytic point of view. In *The cry for help*, ed. N.L. Farberow and E.S. Shneidman, pp. 181-92. New York: McGraw-Hill.

Lidz, T. 1968. *The person: His development throughout the life cycle*. New York: Basic Books.

Seiden, R.H. 1969. *Suicide among youth*. Bulletin of Suicidology (Supplement).

Teicher, J.D., and Jacobs, J. 1966. Adolescents who attempt suicide. *American Journal of Psychiatry* 122:1248-57.

The Analysis of an Adolescent at Risk

With Comments on the Relation between Psychopathology and Technique

Moses Laufer   *London*

INTRODUCTION

In my experience of the psychoanalytic treatment of adolescents, I have frequently been faced with the need to deal with specific actions or acting out behaviour of a very serious nature. At times these actions have endangered patients' lives or have at least placed them in serious danger of harm to themselves; or the adolescent has done things which have endangered the future of his treatment. From my contact with a number of colleagues who treat adolescents psychoanalytically, such actions or acting out behaviour are not at all uncommon during the treatment of *seriously disturbed* adolescents. In certain circumstances, it may mean that the psychoanalyst is then faced with the need to ''do something'' about this specific action, otherwise the adolescent may actually be endangered in some way. In other less serious circumstances, it is the treatment itself that may end as the result of certain actions. I am referring to such behaviour as the extensive taking of drugs, or attempted suicide, or becoming pregnant, or of involving oneself in actions which could result in legal proceedings.

A hesitation I have in discussing some of the technical problems encountered in the treatment of such seriously disturbed adolescents is that it may create the impression that "management" of one kind or another is sufficient to overcome some of the very difficult problems with which the analyst is faced. I do not believe this. A number of authors have described the varied problems facing the analyst of adolescents (Blos, 1966; Frankl and Hellman, 1962; Geleerd, 1961), and some of these authors have suggested guides which may be used temporarily in the adaptation of classical technique in handling specific problems in treatment (see especially Eissler, 1958). I, too, have found it appropriate at times to use explanation, clarification of aims, and sometimes to actually intervene in the day-to-day lives of some adolescents who may be at risk or in danger of some kind. Many adolescents in treatment are in the midst of a serious crisis in their present lives, often with the need to make decisions affecting their future education and future work. Sometimes, this kind of concern by the adolescent about an immediate crisis can mistakenly be seen as a resistance, and the significance of the crisis can be lost. These problems seem to be shared by many adolescents in treatment, and temporary adaptation of classical technique is appropriate here in dealing with a crisis in the adolescent's life.

However, in her paper "Adolescence," Anna Freud (1958) warns against oversimplifying the problems encountered in the treatment of adolescents, and she states the following:

- Experience has taught us to take a serious view of such major and repeated inadequacies of the analytic technique. They cannot be explained away by individual characteristics of the patients under treatment nor by any accidental or environmental factors which run counter to it. Nor can they be overcome simply by increased effort, skill and tact on the part of the analyst. They have to be taken as indications that something in the inner structure of the disturbances themselves differs markedly from the pattern of those illnesses for which the analytic technique has been devised originally and to which it is most frequently applied. We have to gain insight into these divergencies of pathology before we are in a position to revise our technique (pp. 261-62).

The adolescent patient I am describing in this paper shares one important characteristic with some other adolescent patients—a characteristic which can be used as a sign that it may be necessary for the analyst to intervene in the adolescent's behaviour. This characteristic can often be detected early in one's therapeutic contact with the adolescent. In the course of the analysis, it becomes clear that the adolescent, himself, is not able to stop doing certain things of a serious and sometimes dangerous nature. During treatment, it then becomes possible to recognise that *this behaviour is equivalent to the repetitive living out in the outside world of a specific fantasy or fantasies, and that this is something which these kinds of adolescents feel compelled to do*. It also becomes clear that the more they live out these fantasies, the more anxious and disorganised they seem to become. As treatment progresses, these adolescents then begin to acknowledge that *interpretation of the meaning of the specific fantasy or fantasies does not help them to stop putting certain of these fantasies into action*. But the dilemma is that the success or failure of treatment may depend just on this ability to isolate these fantasies and to be able to bring them into the analysis for understanding and working through. Reality factors, such as the real danger to themselves of some of their actions, do not seem to have any impact on them. In such circumstances, it then becomes important for the analyst temporarily to adopt certain measures which could be described as "parameters" (Eissler, 1958), that is, to place clearly defined limits on the adolescent's behaviour. The analyst must then, through his intervention, bring this material into the treatment. However, such an intervention must never be simply an external matter which the analyst superimposes; it must be something which is understood by the patient, and which is experienced by the patient as being necessary and of potential help to the progress of the treatment. Such intervention took place during the treatment of Jane, and I will present some of the analytic material presently.

The timing of these interventions is therefore crucial. I do not think they would be of any use if they were brought into the treatment at a time when the adolescent did not feel he had a relationship to the analyst. It is important to wait until the adolescent acknowledges that his pathology and behaviour are interfering seriously with his life, and for him to begin to see that his need for certain forms of action or of acting out is a serious problem in his life. It would be an error to intervene unless the intervention can make affective sense to the adolescent. The intervention must, therefore, come at a time when the adolescent can allow himself to use the analyst temporarily as an auxiliary ego or auxiliary superego.

One danger, of course, about intervening is that the treatment may then become sexualised: it is as if the adolescent may feel that he has been able to force the analyst to become the controlling and the punishing superego and, in this way, that he is forcing the analyst to fit into his fantasy of being passively subdued by the analyst. The sexualisation of the treatment can be a very serious resistance, but this is nevertheless more manageable than the continuous loss of the content of the fantasy through the adolescent's actions outside the sessions, as well as the loss of the affect attached to these actions.

The adolescents whom I am describing—one of whom is Jane, and whose clinical material will follow—are usually very vulnerable people, some with histories of attempted suicide, self-mutilation, extensive taking of drugs, promiscuity. Because of the vulnerability of these adolescents, the analyst may be hesitant to disturb the treatment, and may want to avoid any unnecessary "crises". Some of these adolescents unconsciously know also that their vulnerability frightens people and makes people kind and cautious towards them. A tendency could be for the analyst to want to avoid any of the adolescent's negative transference reactions, partly because of the belief that taking up the negative transference might provoke the adolescent to break off treatment or to act out in some other way. But this avoidance by the analyst produces greater anxiety in the adolescent because the adolescent will unconsciously sense that the analyst, too, is frightened. This, itself, then results in a greater need on the part of the adolescent to act out this aspect of the transference. This acting out of the transference can then become confused in the adolescent's mind with other forms of "uncontrolled" behaviour, and he will become even more frightened by his actions.

Those adolescents to whom I am referring feel temporarily unable to stop some of their behaviour without the analyst's help, and this feeling of being unable to stop exists well before treatment has begun. The treatment may highlight the need of the adolescent to repeat certain forms of behaviour which are, in fact, part of the pathology, but the treatment itself does not produce this need to repeat certain behaviour. It is only after the analyst places defined limits on some specific behaviour of the adolescent that the adolescent feels able to begin to gain some insight into the meaning of those fantasies which *compel* him to behave in certain ways. With some adolescents whom I have treated by psychoanalysis, I have noticed that treatment really begins to get underway only after these fantasies are "pulled" into the analysis. Once these actions do come under analytic scrutiny, *it becomes obvious that the fantasies which these adolescents are compelled to live out in a repetitive way are the adolescent's central masturbation fantasy.* It also becomes clear during treatment that these adolescents, although they may be able to masturbate, are not able to use masturbation as a "trial action," that is, as an autoerotic activity which helps to integrate regressive fantasies as a part of the effort to achieve genital dominance (Laufer, 1968).

Other than this intervention is a very defined area of such patients' lives, I think it is possible and advisable to use classical analytic technique. Unnecessary intervention confuses the adolescent and distorts the development of the transference. The confusion lies in the fact that unnecessary intervention makes it impossible for the adolescent to differentiate between behaviour which he feels compelled to live out and behaviour which is specifically related to the treatment and to the present state of the transference.

CASE MATERIAL

I have known Jane since the age of 14, seeing her irregularly up to the age of 17, and then in psychoanalytic treatment for the past two years. When Jane was first brought to me by her parents, she was attending a school some distance from my consulting room, and her visits to me meant a two-hour train ride. I arranged to see her irregularly because of the distance involved, but I was concerned from the start because of her general manner. She always smiled and seemed especially polite and understanding. Her parents had been worried about her isolation, her depression, and her unpredictable moods. They had separated five years earlier, but kept contact with each other about Jane's behaviour and about their concern that she was very unhappy. Her behaviour at her school worried the teachers and me, but all I could do was to be available irregularly, or whenever Jane felt like telephoning me. She and I agreed that this kind of contact would continue until she was ready to leave her present school.

When it was time for Jane to decide about her further education, she said that she was thinking of applying to a university out of London so that she could "get away from everything." By this time she knew that I took a serious view of her disturbance. I questioned whether to be in a city where she could not have intensive treatment might not be a mistake because I felt that her disturbance was such that, without help now, she would remain a very unhappy person. I said that I thought she should have intensive treatment and I, therefore, suggested that she apply to a college in London. She did not decide about this for some months, saying that she could not be sure whether intensive treatment would really help or whether it would destroy her. During this period of my contact with Jane, I did not know what this fear really referred to and, because of this, I felt it would be more appropriate simply to say that I was worried about her and that she needed to have treatment. It was only much later in her analysis that we could make sense of this fear of being destroyed and of her wish to get me to take over the responsibility for this decision. This will be discussed in the paper. She finally decided to apply to a university in the centre of the city so that intensive treatment could be undertaken.

Jane was actually most keen and relieved to be able to come to treatment on a regular basis. She had become very frightened at school when she had what she described as an "hysterical attack" on a school outing—crying, shouting, demanding to be taken back to school. She was very worried about being "sexually abnormal" which to her meant that she might be lesbian; she was unable to have any close relationships with boys; and she felt compelled to masturbate, "the little man in me tells me to do it, and it is as if I just have to." The details of her fears and the content of her masturbation fantasies will be discussed within the context of the treatment material.

Throughout Jane's treatment I have been concerned about the extent of her psychopathology. Fifteen months ago she attempted suicide (after having been in analysis for about seven months), and for about three months after the suicide attempt she showed behaviour which made me wonder whether there were psychotic areas in her functioning which were of such a nature that treatment might be severely hindered.

I should like to concentrate on some of the events and the treatment material which preceded and followed Jane's suicide attempt, and to discuss how I dealt with some of the acting out which followed the suicide attempt. She had been going out with a man, Bill, aged 25. He was described by her as a depressed, ineffectual person who behaved as if he were grateful to her for allowing him to be her boy friend. They had intercourse quite regularly, but Jane was never able to have a climax, this being a constant source of worry to her, and making her feel that it was a confirmation of her abnormality. More specifically, it seemed to me that she was repeatedly being faced with her preference for masturbation, when she could experience in fantasy the idea of being humiliated, overwhelmed, and sometimes raped.

Before she started her relationship with Bill, Jane had been promiscuous for about a year. She would have intercourse with people in a rather indiscriminate way and then would hate herself for this, saying that she was just a "slut" and "should be dead." But intercourse never did what she hoped it would, and she began to masturbate in a rather compulsive way. The effort at that point in the analysis to understand the fantasy during masturbation was not at all successful; and I learned only later about that part of the fantasy she never described when she talked about her masturbation. She told me that she would imagine, in masturbation, that somebody (she was not sure who) was masturbating her furiously and that the only important thing was that she must have a climax. I learned later that the masturbation was often preceded by eating, some drinking, or by reading a novel.

The guilt which Jane experienced as the result of her masturbation was such that she found it extremely difficult to do any of her college work, or to concentrate on anything other than the most mundane kinds of chores. She felt that she was completely paralysed by this need to try to disprove her abnormality and that everything else took second place. But I think that she was referring to something related to the treatment and to a limitation on her behaviour which I had placed on her a short time after her analytic treatment had begun. It was this specific limitation, I think, which made it possible for her to be confronted with the masturbation fantasy and with the fact that she had to live out this specific fantasy in a compelling way. I am referring to the following: When she was at her school some distance from my consulting room, she often would hitchhike into the city. She is an attractive girl, and she was often given a ride by somebody who might then want her telephone number or who might try to pet or have intercourse with her. She never permitted intercourse with any of these men, but she often would allow them to become sexually aroused through petting. A number of times she was given rides by men who threatened to beat her up or to harm her in some way. I became very concerned because this behaviour of hers had a compelling quality to it, and because in reality, she was placing herself in serious danger.

By this time I had become aware that Jane was, through her hitchhiking, living out her central masturbation fantasy. I had tried many times previously to convey to her some of the meaning of the hitchhiking, but she invariably had found reasons to "accept" an offer of a ride. She had, by then, begun to recognise herself that she could not give this up, but she denied any anxiety about it. I told her that it seemed to me that, for some unknown reason, she could not give up hitchhiking, and that I was very concerned for her safety. I also said that, unless she stopped hitchhiking, we would not be able to understand what was forcing her to behave in this way, and that the treatment would be interfered with, and I added: "It is for this reason that I think you should not hitchhike any longer." Jane was both furious and relieved. I was aware that such a decision might interfere with the normal course of the treatment, but I felt that we had reached a point in the analysis where Jane could see that she could not stop this behaviour on her own.

The central masturbation fantasy to which I am referring is the following:

> She is being chased, and is then caught, by a man who looks completely unconcerned and who has no feelings at all. This man then gets her to do all kinds of things for him, in a slavelike way, and then he proceeds to excite her sexually. He is in complete control of himself and of what is going on. She submits to his demands for sexual activity, but the fantasy then ends abruptly just before they have intercourse.

I call this her central masturbation fantasy, but in fact in masturbation she did not consciously have this fantasy. It was usually lived out in some way in her relationship with people, as, for example, in the hitchhiking. The fantasy during masturbation was much more neutral and, as she said, much more "clinical," that is, she did it "just to get physical relief."

Jane constantly complained of her relationship to Bill, saying that he humiliated himself in her eyes, that he was not strong enough and that she could get him to do anything she asked. In the transference, she constantly tried to put me into the position of the man in her masturbation fantasy by insisting that I show my strength, and by saying that I did not care for her if I only talked and did not take any active part in stopping her from doing things. On Mondays she would describe her weekend behaviour with Bill, and she demanded that I do something to control her, saying that I was stupid to go on treating her. Why did I not stop treatment? She was no good, worthless, dirty, and I was no better if I listened to her and if I allowed her to come to see me each day. (This had been of much concern to me when I had decided earlier to stop the hitchhiking, that is, that I might fit into her fantasy of being the brutal, cold person who forced her to submit to me. But the reality was of such a nature that I felt I must take that chance, and then bring this ensuing transference factor into the treatment for analysis and working through.)

Up to the time preceding her suicide attempt, we had recognised Jane's fear of her abnormality, her worry about being lesbian, her belief that she had in some way been responsible for her parents' separation, and her great discomfort in being with other people of her own age. She felt convinced that masturbation confirmed that there was something seriously wrong with her mentally, but at the same time she felt unable to "forget about it, or at least not have to go on doing it." These problems were discussed a great deal in treatment. But any mention by me of her wish that I declare my love for her, or any reference to the extent of the destructive capacity she felt she had inside herself, were completely rejected —to the point where she told me that I was accusing her of "thinking about things which don't exist," that I did not really show interest in her, and that she sometimes wanted to run away and die. While in the sessions, she often talked in a very quiet voice, smiled in a rather waxlike way, and held tightly to her feelings. But outside the sessions, she often argued with her boy friend, cried and screamed, would not talk for hours at a time, and would at times stay in her room and not allow anybody to come in.

A fortnight before her suicide attempt, she became extremely anxious about her relationship to Bill, as well as about her repeated masturbation. She continued to have intercourse with Bill, but complained that it was all useless, that she did not really feel that intercourse satisfied her, but at the same time she could not give it up. If she did, she would be left on her own and to herself, and she would just go on trying to excite herself, and that would be horrible and abnormal. Interpretation at this point did not seem to have any effect. She continued to become increasingly agitated and said that she just could not stop masturbating. Coming to treatment was no use, she said, because she was here only for under an hour and she was then left on her own for the rest of the day. Her concern during masturbation at this time was to achieve a climax: "I don't care what I think about, I just want to get it over with. Don't you understand? If I don't get it over with, I'll go crazy." She felt sure that she was becoming very abnormal; nor did intercourse with Bill change this feeling.

At college, she had met an older woman student, and they had become friendly. This woman obligingly told Jane that masturbation was a very good way of ridding oneself of tension, and Jane took this remark as further permission to go on masturbating. The result, however, was not temporary relief, but much greater anxiety and a feeling that she was now free to lose complete control of herself. To Jane, this simply exaggerated the extent to which she felt that her body was her enemy and that one way to rid herself of that dirty, horrible thing which made her feel lesbian was to kill it. When this older woman friend (who represented Jane's relationship to her lonely and isolated mother) told Jane to "have a go," that is, to masturbate, Jane felt excited by this kind of closeness. Interpretation of her wish for closeness to this woman and to her mother made her silent and frightened. All she could say was, "I hate Bill, but I must not let go." At the same time, she accused me of not caring because I had not tried to stop her masturbation.

The day before the suicide attempt, Jane came to her session saying that she felt she was losing control of herself, and that suddenly everything had gone out of her life. She giggled when she said that she had thought of hitchhiking "somewhere" and of how nice it would be if a man with a lovely sports car were to give her a ride "somewhere." She had "almost decided" to try and get a ride but she did not know what made her change her mind. She did not want Bill, yet she could not be rid of him; she did not want to masturbate, yet she had to go on doing it. She began to weep very quietly, still trying to maintain control. I continued to try to get to what I thought was now the core of her anxiety, that is, that she regarded her thoughts as now very abnormal and that she was ashamed of what she felt and thought. When I referred to the "little man in her who tells her to do it,'' she simply said that she could not talk about "certain things.'' (It was only after some months following her suicide attempt that she·talked of a part of her thoughts that nobody must take away from her. She did not know what this was, but she felt there was a part of her mind that nobody could or would get to; it was hers, and she could not give that part away.)

Jane was at home alone when she took an overdose of pills and she was found some hours later by her boy friend. By coincidence, she was admitted to a hospital where an analytic colleague is a senior member of the hospital staff. It was two days before she fully regained consciousness. I visited her there once where she had an analytic session, after which she came on her own, or was brought, to her sessions from hospital. This arrangement lasted for nearly three months. She stayed in hospital a total of five months.[1] During the period immediately following her suicide attempt, some of her behaviour in the hospital and with Bill made me wonder whether she might be psychotic.[2] Jane was very difficult at the hospital, was often sullen, argued with the other patients, sometimes broke dishes, and once disappeared from the hospital for some hours before she was found sitting by the bank of a river. When asked by the nurse why she had stormed out of the hospital (something she did on two occasions in treatment), she said that she had had an argument with another girl in the ward, and she had felt that one way of settling it all was to jump into the river. She became involved in fights in the ward, slapped some of the male patients who "keep on trying to touch me,'' and was generally unpredictable and extremely moody.

Her sessions, during this first period following her suicide attempt, were almost totally disorganised. Interpretation of her defensive behaviour, that is, in relation to her fear that she was abnormal, or to her worry that she might really kill herself, or to her fear that she would attack her mother, helped her very slightly. But she remained extremely anxious, and in general there was very little change. She often cried now in her sessions, pulling at her hair, and saying repeatedly, "I *must* die. It will never be right. I must die." She explained this as a feeling that nothing would be right until she did die. I decided that I had to make my position clear at this point, that is, that I was in reality not able to stop her from killing herself. I felt now that, whatever the interpretation might be of her present behaviour, it was equally important to bring the reality into the treatment. I explained that I could help her, but that I could do so only if she felt she wanted to go on living. I stated that if she wanted to kill herself I could not stop her, and I reminded her that her wish to die and her earlier suicide attempt was a sign of illness. It was with her illness that I could help her, but I could do this only if she had decided that she wanted help. She was furious, but at the same time she seemed to calm down.

From this time, Jane began to bring material to her sessions which was much more related to her feeling that she was going completely mad and that she was on the verge of what she described as "disintegration." She could not describe it in any other way, she said. She felt terrified of that "core" to which she had referred earlier, and which she felt she could not let anybody get to. She repeated often that her pathology was in this core (meaning a part of her thinking which she had never been able to share with anybody). The trouble was, she said, that she did not really know what this core was all about. She felt that she was dirty and useless, and that she just had to die. Nothing else could take the place of death.[3]

It was at this juncture that I reminded Jane of an incident which she had referred to as "that time," but which she could not mention unless "I have to," an incident which she felt she had to, somehow, eliminate from "my body." Soon after her analytic treatment had begun, she had met a man who had taken her to his home. There he masturbated her with a tubelike object. She had felt completely "crazy" when this happened—she had enjoyed it as well as feeling disgusted by it. She was convinced that it was only through death that she could be rid of this experience "from my body." There was no other way; death was the only way that this experience could be "ended once and for all." Then all the secrets would be dead, too. But she could not define these secrets—she did not know what they were, but she felt they were always there to be hidden from herself as well as from others.

Jane now described how terrified she had been of treatment, that is, of finding out that she was irreversibly abnormal. She could not tell me things freely because this would mean that she had given in to me. And if she gave in to me, "then it means that I will have to tell you that I care. People think that things don't matter to me, that I'm cold, or that I'm satisfied with everything." She suddenly then became silent. Before the end of that session, she began to cry and could then say that she was convinced I would not be able to help her. She could not be sure whether I liked her or despised her; whatever she did, it did not seem to frighten me. She felt safe because of this, but at the same time I might despise her for such behaviour. In fact, she was referring to some of her recent behaviour in hospital—fighting with the other patients, drinking wine and "making myself stupid," and spending much time with a young married woman (also a patient) who had violent outbursts of anger.

The crisis seemed very serious at this point, and I was unsure about Jane's prognosis or, for that matter, about her day-to-day behaviour. I felt that, technically, it was important at this point not to try to use reconstruction, but instead to locate some of the content of her daydreams, as well as of her other extreme behaviour. It seemed to me that reconstruction at this moment in the crisis might temporarily alleviate the anxiety but that, on the other hand, it might also produce greater anxiety. I tried, therefore, to concentrate on the details of her present behaviour in hospital: when she went to sleep, what she ate, how she spent her day, what she thought about while in the ward, what she read, who she talked to, and so on. It was from these details that I could begin to understand the extent to which Jane felt bewildered by what had gone on recently in her life, and the extent to which she felt that she could "lose control" at any time.

She came to her session one day, and began by saying that she had again thought "I must die." She felt she must talk to me about it. While on the bus on the way to her session, she had felt crazy again. In the waiting room, she did not know what to do—should she sit, or stand, read, look out of the window. Nothing had felt right. It had felt as if she had to do something. She had looked at her fingernails while waiting for me. She had thought it would be nice to tear my skin with her fingernails, or maybe she should do it to somebody else. I was so detached and all I wanted to do was understand; maybe tearing my skin would break me down? That would be nice. She then felt very frightened. Silence. She then pulled at her hair and began to scream, saying "I don't know what it is. I really must die. Please help me." Then silence again. She reacted with astonishment when she remembered that she had awakened during the night from a nightmare. She had completely forgotten about this; it only came back now. She could not recall the details. But it felt horrible. Now she felt crazy. The nightmare made her feel crazy. She then remembered the following dream: Jane is being loved by, and is loving, another girl. She thought it would be nice to masturbate this girl and to be masturbated by her. She couldn't remember anything else about this "nightmare," except that the nurse woke her up while she was dreaming. She had felt terrible. She had not been able to fall asleep for a long time because of the thoughts about the girl. When she had awakened, she did not remember this dream at all. She only went on feeling terrible, and thinking that she must die, that there was no hope, that she was no good, and that she would never get out of hospital.

Jane then recalled that on the previous evening she had felt very miserable. The ward had seemed very depressing. She had gone out and had bought some wine. She had known that the hospital prohibited this, but she had not cared. She and another patient (the young married woman referred to earlier) had begun to drink the wine. As she drank, she had felt a sensation in her vagina, as if she wanted something to happen. Silence. She then thought how nice it might be to touch this other patient, to hold each other, and perhaps to be loved by this patient. "I love and I hate her. When I was getting drunk, I wanted her to hold me and I wanted to hold her." The dream was awful. It made her feel hopeless and dangerous.

She remembered how she and her younger sister used to sleep in the same room as children. Sometimes they would sleep in the same bed, and when it was dark they would even hold each other. They had looked very much alike. Sometimes, as little children, they would "tell" each other when to start masturbating. This meant that they had a word which meant that one had started to masturbate; and this then meant that the other would start. When Bill (her boy friend) had intercourse with her, he didn't seem to know that what she really wanted was to be held, just held and made safe, nothing else. She used to hate intercourse because it always reminded her that she was abnormal; she couldn't have a climax, and she felt so dirty all the time. That would never change. But she had to go on having intercourse because otherwise she would just want to be with girls, and that would make her want to die.

When her father had visited her in hospital the other day, all she had been able to do was to cry. She liked him less now than she used to, and she didn't know whether she blamed him for what she did. It was so confusing: she felt so abnormal and so lonely, and she did not know whether it would help to blame anybody. But at the same time, when she thought of dying, she sometimes thought that she could in this way make others feel that it was their fault. But that wasn't the real reason for wanting to die. It was because she had to get rid of all those secrets in her body.

When I said that, from the dream, it seemed as if she felt that she preferred to be held rather than to have intercourse, and that this feeling of wanting to be held was for her a proof of her abnormality, she recalled how she had wanted to touch the woman patient the previous night. She "almost did it, but I don't know what made me stop." When I said that her bewilderment and her feeling that she must die was partially her way of punishing her body for wanting such things, and that it was as if she really now wanted to be held by her mother, Jane replied that when she was "coming round after I took the overdose, my mother was sitting by my bed. My mother told me the other day that I said to her now she and I were closer to each other than ever before. I hated her for telling me that. And I forgot it until now." But now she felt as if she could fight this just a little, maybe she didn't have to be lesbian; maybe it was more that she hated Bill for being weak and so dependent. Her father had once cried when he and her mother were thinking of separating, and she had hated him too. But when he left, she felt as if she herself had really driven him out of the house; it was as if she wanted to be alone with her mother, but at the same time she knew that her father was now strong.

She hated me too for that, but she also didn't hate me. When I came to the hospital to see her, she remembered thinking that I might look frightened, but I didn't look that way. "I thought you might be angry with me for letting you down. But I remember that you said you couldn't stop me from killing myself if I wanted to do that. It felt as if you were telling me to die. But I knew what you meant. Will I get you to throw me out? How can you take this from me? Why don't you do what you should? You should say you don't want to see me anymore." When I answered that she needed me now to confirm for her the feeling that she was worthless, and that she could drive me away as she felt she had driven her father away, she did not reply. She then was silent for the few remaining minutes of the session. When she left, she was crying. As she walked out of the consulting room, she said, "I'll be all right. Don't worry."

I had previously interpreted, a number of times, Jane's attachment to her sister as representing Jane's wish to be close to her mother and to be held by her. But Jane had said that she never felt this "even though it sounds right." This dream seemed to enable her to begin to bring material which was related to her "secrets," and to her feeling that there was a "core" which nobody, not even herself, could get to. But she also now spent a great deal of time being silent. Sometimes she would leave at the end of a session feeling very angry, and at other times she would smile and say goodbye. Her silences showed the extent of her fear that I might break her down, and also her feeling that she could come to a session at times and be left alone with me without having to be the "best patient." After she had understood part of the foregoing dream, she felt that it was less necessary to say "I must die." She now changed this to: "I think I should die." She said that if she were "really mad," or if she "might be mad" in the future, then it would be better to be dead. She had seen some of the more ill patients, and they were so miserable. What was the purpose of living like that? She might as well finish it off, and everybody, including me, might be relieved. But at the same time, she felt slightly more hopeful. It was as if the dream had devastated her, but it hadn't really, and that made her more hopeful. But now she felt frightened when she went to bed, because she might have another dream like that, and this would be horrible. She asked the ward doctor for sleeping pills, and she said that the pills were her way of making sure that she was not awakened by something from inside attacking her as it did in the dream.

For weeks Jane was unable to fall asleep even after having taken the sleeping pills. I concentrated during this time on her feeling that she would be overwhelmed by her inside attacker and by the abnormal part of herself. This seemed to help. She began to ask during her sessions whether it might be a good idea to "risk" going to bed without taking the sleeping pills. At this point, I did not interpret the obvious transference meaning that she felt more trust in me and that I was now helping her. When she began to take fewer sleeping pills, she sometimes spent part of the night awake and thinking that she must not give in to the abnormal part of herself. She risked having "horrible dreams" because she thought that these would help us understand the "crazy part" of herself. But she remained frightened because she thought that if she did not sleep she would then have to go on masturbating, and that would be "the end."

After approximately six weeks in hospital, Jane felt able to return to the university for part of each day. At first she felt ashamed of being ill. She thought of leaving the university and finding work "where I can be away from normal people." But she felt relieved and less vulnerable when she became friendly with another female student who herself had thought of suicide and who was now very depressed and unable to keep up with her university work. Soon after her return to the university, Jane "suddenly found that I could tell Bill that I didn't want him." It was as if she could give him up and, if necessary, risk "going back to masturbating all the time." To her this meant that she was running the risk of becoming seriously ill again. She was also worried that she might want to start hitchhiking again, and perhaps get a man to do something to her, that is, to harm her in some way. This was her constant daydream—of being chased, caught, overpowered, and humiliated in some way. She said that she knew that she had agreed not to hitchhike.

Jane brought her daydream now into the transference through her very lengthy silences, and through her refusal to tell me what she was thinking about. At first this made her anxious and very angry. When I interpreted her present silence as being equivalent to getting me to run after her, catch her, and force her to talk, that is, of wanting to satisfy the wish in the daydream here in the session, she could admit that "when I am silent I sometimes feel excited, and I wait for you to force me." The rape fantasy was obvious, and when I said that now she wanted me forcibly to get into her, she said it was just that which had made her feel most excited sexually in her relationship with Bill. She used to walk about in the nude in the presence of her father, and she used to hope that she might be able to get him excited so that he would do something to her. She remembered how, when her parents separated, she used to visit her father. Once she had stayed the weekend with him. She had got into his bed in the nude and had slept near him. She had hoped he would do something to her, but when he had told her to put on some clothes, she had felt despair and had thought then that "everything was hopeless." She used to try to "fool him in all kinds of ways": she would leave the lavatory door unlocked; she would call to him when she was having a bath, but it did not work. He "never gave in." Jane's silences in her sessions contained this theme of fooling me, of withholding things which she felt I should know, or of talking in generalisations so that I would not be sure of what she meant. To her, fooling me was equivalent now to having a secret, a "core that nobody could get to."

I shall now proceed to a later period in Jane's analysis. After she had been out of hospital for nearly six months, she met a student, Mark, who very quickly became her boy friend. Until that time she had spent a great deal of time alone; or she had gone out with boys and sometimes had had intercourse. Mark had known that she had attempted suicide. He felt that her illness was now past and thought there was no need for her to continue with her daily treatment. She told me of this and said that she, too, had thought of coming less often but was frightened of giving me up because I was the only person who was not afraid of her and who also kept her "in control." She was sure that she would "go wild again if I stop coming here." During those times when she was getting on well with her boy friend she was able to talk to me about what was going on and how she felt, and we seemed able to continue to try to understand her feeling that she must die. If she argued with Mark, or if she felt that I did not like her, she would say that she was again thinking of suicide. I interpreted the threat, the feeling of hopelessness, the attack on her body, or the attack on the internalised parent. But aside from my actual interpretations, I made it clear that I could not stop her. She had become familiar now with the probability that her thoughts about killing herself were brought on by some "abnormal thoughts," that is, by some thought or action which she considered to be a sign of abnormality. When she could tell me about the fellatio/cunnilingus between herself and Mark, she again could stop threatening that she might kill herself.

This recognition that the immediate anxiety about her abnormality and the thought that she "must die" were linked to a thought or action, which she considered abnormal, was an important insight. This also helped her to withstand some of the pressure from Mark to attend her sessions less often. She said, "It feels a bit untrue that maybe something can change." In some ways, it felt safer to be ill—then everybody could say, "She's not well, don't be angry with her." Her parents had had trouble in the past; sometimes she even wondered whether there might be something wrong with her mother. She remembered when her mother had told her, about two or three years previously, to "have a go," that is, to feel free to masturbate, when she felt tense. Jane then wondered at times whether her mother really wanted to force her to masturbate.

"Permission is all right, but does she know what she is saying when she says such a thing?"

It was within this context that my earlier request that she stop hitchhiking could again be brought into the treatment. She had previously mentioned her wish to hitchhike "just for the fun of it," but she was able to stop herself from doing this. Now she wanted to try again to see if she could be in control of what might occur. When she said this and I did not immediately reply, she asked why I did not care any longer. What had she done? What was the use then? Why get better if it didn't matter to me? Here I made the link again with part of her daydream: of feeling forced to do certain things, of being chased, and now of wanting again to try to get me to show her that I was the one in control, but at the same time the one who was detached. I also said that she knew now that she did not have to hitchhike, she had the control; but what was important for her now was for me to show that I wanted her to be loyal only to me, that is, to keep her body only for me. She reacted to this by being silent, and then she began to cry. I said nothing when she cried. Before she left she said, "When you said that, you took it away from me. Now I feel you don't want me."

The next day Jane arrived saying, "I'm sorry about yesterday. I didn't want to be upset, and I didn't want to upset you. It was only a bit of a shock to hear you say what I've been thinking." When I said that she had to make amends, to try to be my best patient, and to make sure that neither of us felt any anger at any time, she replied, "Drop dead! You and your wife. You can both drop dead. I'll do what I want. You just wait and see. You said you can't stop me from dying. Well, you won't stop me!" I replied, "You're frightened of me now. But I haven't changed from yesterday. I wonder what has happened since you were here yesterday?" She was silent for nearly twenty minutes. She then said she had been thinking of all the things that she was not going to talk about, of having masturbated after intercourse with Mark, and of not caring any longer what was going to happen. She was frightened to tell me that after intercourse with Mark, she often had to masturbate because she could not have a climax during intercourse. This humiliated her and at the same time "it means we're back to my keeping secrets from everybody. Mark doesn't know about this, and I think he's stupid because he doesn't know." I said, "I wonder what I don't know, and I wonder why I have to force you to tell me?" "I'm going to kill myself. That's what you don't know. There's no hope. I know it." On the previous day she had been with a girl friend from the university and she had thought that this girl had nice breasts—nicer than her own—and she had felt envious. She had wanted to touch them. When she had come home, she had wanted to have intercourse immediately with Mark, but even that had not helped. After intercourse, she had looked at herself and had felt that she did not look nice enough. I reminded her of what we had talked about in the previous session. She said that she had completely forgotten that she felt she was not good enough for me, that I did not want her. "Anyway, you know about all my dirt, so you wouldn't want me. I'm surprised you still see me, after what you know." I said, "You mean you are surprised that you haven't driven me away."

When she came on the following Monday, Jane told me that she had been to a party on the previous Saturday night and had got drunk. Mark had not minded too much because he, too, had too much to drink. She had made a fool of herself, and she did not care. Well, that was not true, because she really cared very much. When she awoke on the Sunday morning, she felt that she had humiliated herself and that Mark too must have felt humiliated because of the way she had behaved. The acting out of part of the transference could be interpreted at this point, that is, that her humiliation was in relation to me and her behaviour at the party was her need to live out a part of the daydream which she felt she could not be rid of. When I reminded her of her earlier efforts to break down her father by presenting herself in the nude, and feeling rejected by him when he did not respond as she had hoped he would, she replied, "You don't care what I do, do you? If you did care, maybe you would tell me not to get drunk?''

For some time, the themes of humiliating herself, of fooling people, and of having a secret from everybody, remained the central ones. Jane's guilt was enormous, and the combination of this guilt with her feeling that she would "go on being abnormal" (feel attracted at times to girls, prefer masturbation to intercourse, and be unable to have a climax during intercourse) continued to make her feel that she must not give up "the final weapon" (as she described it) of being able to kill herself. Her sudden outbursts in the sessions, her crying and screaming in some sessions, followed by very quiet speech, were part of her fantasy that I was the only person who could give her a climax and, in that sense, enable her to become normal or, at least, to forget "those secrets that I can't get rid of.''

This primal scene material has now dominated Jane's analysis for many months. Reconstruction has been limited up to this point, but there has obviously been an important change in Jane's relationship to her illness and in her feeling that she is the victim of both her daydreams and her abnormal thoughts. She still reports that she is often frightened of falling asleep, that is, of being overwhelmed by frightening thoughts which, in waking life, she can temporarily control. Although her fear of being abnormal is still certainly present, she seems to have less need to feel that she "must die." Some of this improvement or, at least, this lessened vulnerability to her need to humiliate herself and then attack her body, was shown in a dream which she recently reported. This dream was, in some ways, similar to the one described earlier, but Jane's ability to deal with the enormous anxiety aroused by this dream was now quite different. In this dream, Jane was being masturbated by a school friend. The school friend, a girl, suddenly withdrew her finger as Jane was being sexually aroused. From Jane's associations to this dream, we could again make the link to her feeling that she and her sister were masturbating each other and that she might prefer this to intercourse. Again we could also make the link to Jane's feeling, during masturbation, that she was really being held by her mother and that this was how she imagined the perfect primal scene. The difference now was that Jane seemed much more able to deal *actively* with the enormous anxiety which had been aroused by this dream. She still referred to it as "a nightmare," but she was much less disorganised by it. She could say now that she knew that she would not masturbate whenever she was alone, and that now she was beginning to feel able to "feel alone without feeling also that I must die." (Jane was referring to the time, earlier in her treatment, when she masturbated often. Then she felt "out of control," and she remembered correctly that this extensive masturbation was a signal that she was then becoming much more seriously disturbed.)

Jane's analytic treatment is still continuing. She and I both know that she is still very vulnerable and that there is much to understand in her behaviour and pathology. But, at the same time, she feels much more able to make the effort to overcome "that part of myself which is abnormal." The secrets are still there, or at least Jane feels they are. The idea of killing her body as a way of ridding herself of these secrets seems to have decreased.

COMMENT

The material which I have reported in this paper is only a fragment of Jane's analysis. I have chosen certain material in order to discuss some aspects of her pathology as well as the relation between this pathology and some technical problems encountered in the treatment. I have not included that material which might be considered part of normal adolescence and which, therefore, would not be used by me to understand Jane's pathology. In other words, the analytic work was consistently directed toward the pathology and did not bring in for understanding that part of Jane's behaviour which represented the normal developmental stresses of adolescence.

The problem of "management" or of "setting certain limits" in Jane's treatment was very restricted. In looking back at the progress of her treatment, it seems that the restriction on her hitchhiking behaviour made it possible for certain fantasies to come into the treatment for understanding—fantasies which Jane seemed compelled to live out and which otherwise might well have been used in such a way as to endanger her. The setting of this limit was a way of "pulling in" a central masturbation fantasy into the analysis. The treatment of some seriously disturbed adolescents sometimes calls for such temporary parameters. The intervention which I have described has a very specific purpose. But, other than this temporary parameter, classical technique is not only advisable but essential.

NOTES

[1] I arranged with the hospital that she would be discharged when I felt it was all right to do so.

[2] I have been concerned about this with a number of adolescents who have attempted suicide and whose analytic treatment I am following.

[3] At the Centre for the Study of Adolescence, there is a study in progress of adolescents who have attempted suicide. This study consists of eight adolescents in psychoanalytic treatment. Their attitudes to death are of special interest: when they talk of death, it really means killing the body, but not necessarily killing the mind. It is as if, at the time of attempting suicide, they experience their bodies as separate from the rest of themselves and not as belonging to themselves; or death means the removal of consciousness, that is, getting away from their guilt or from their bodies, which they feel to be the source of all the trouble.

BIBLIOGRAPHY

Blos, Peter. 1966. The concept of acting out in relation to the adolescent process. *Journal of the American Academy of Child Psychiatry*, no. 1.

Bissler, K.R. 1958. Notes on problems of technique in the psychoanalytic treatment of adolescents: With special remarks on perversions. *Psychoanalytic Study of the Child* 13:23-54.

Frankl, L., and Hellman, I. 1962. The ego's participation in the therapeutic alliance. *International Journal of Psycho-Analysis* 43:333-37.

Freud, Anna. 1958. Adolescence. *Psychoanalytic Study of the Child* 13:255-78.

Freud, S. 1914. Remembering, repeating, and working-through. *Standard edition* 12:145-56. London: Hogarth Press, 1958.

———. 1917. Mourning and melancholia. *Standard edition* 14:237-60. London: Hogarth Press, 1961.

Friedman, M., Glasser, M., Laufer, E., Laufer, M., and Wohl, M. 1972. Attempted suicide and self-mutilation in adolescence: Some observations from a psychoanalytic research project. *International Journal of Psycho-Analysis*, vol. 53.

Geleerd, E. R. 1961. Some aspects of ego vicissitudes in adolescence. *Journal of the American Psychoanalytic Association* 9:394-405.

Harley, M. 1961. Some observations on the relationship between genitality and structural development at adolescence. *Journal of the American Psychoanalytic Association* 9:434-60.

Laufer, M. 1968. The body image, the function of masturbation and adolescence: Problems of the ownership of the body. *Psychoanalytic Study of the Child* 23:114-37.

Index